MINISTRY OF HEALTH CARE OF THE REPUBLIC OF UZBEKISTAN

URGANCH BRANCH OF TASHKENT MEDICAL ACADEMY

Allanazarov Allanazar Khudashkurovich

Tajitdinova Guzal Gayratovna

SIMULTANEOUS LAPAROSCOPIC OPERATIONS IN PATIENTS WITH HIGH SURGERY RISK

Monograph

Amazon Kindle Direct Publishing
United States of America – 2024

A.K. Allanazarov, G.G. Tajitdinova. Simultaneous laparoscopic operations i
patients with high surgery risk. Monograph

In the monograph, the results of simultaneous laparoscopic operations (SLC
performed in a relatively large volume and wide range of clinical material :
patients with high operational risk were analyzed, as a result of which the:
operations were improved, the most optimal methods were selected and used i
patients with high operational risk. , the results of which were compared and it w:
stated that operational tactics were improved and the most optimal methods we
selected.

This monograph is intended for surgeons with many years of clinic
experience, masters, clinical residents, high-level students of medical universitie
and doctors who are interested in this field.

Simultaneous laparoscopic operations in patients with high surgery risk
monograph / compiled by A.K. Allanazarov, G.G. Tajitdinova. - 2024. – 92 p.

ISBN: 979-88-82964-37-4

CONTENT

ABBREVIATIONS

1. ABP - arterial blood pressure

2. IUD - intrauterine device

3. HD - hypertension disease

4. GIA – sewing machine

5. CT - computed tomography

6. LC - laparoscopic cholecystectomy

7. LA - laparoscopic appendectomy

8. LC - laparoscopic cystectomy

9. LH - laparoscopic hernioplasty

10. LM - laparoscopic myomectomy

11. LESS - laparoscopic elective surgical sterilization

12. WR - Wasserman reaction

13. SLO - Simultaneous laparoscopic operations

14. CSC - chronic stone cholecystitis

15. USE - ultrasound examination

16. CEK – cholecystectomy

17. EGDFS – esophagogastroduodenofibrosiaopia

18. ECG - electrocardiography

19. EcoCG - echocardiography

20. IHD - ischemic heart disease

21. US – ultrasound

22. ASC - acute stone cholecystitis

23. CDAO - co-occurring diseases of abdominal organs

INTRODUCTORY PART

The urgency of the problem. Chronic cholecystitis (CC) is one of the most common diseases in the world today. If this disease occurs in 10-15% of the world's population and this rate doubles on average every 10 years, it is predicted that it will become the main problem in the field of surgical gastroenterology by the second half of the 21st century. [1]

In addition to the high incidence of this disease among the elderly and elderly population, this category of patients has a high risk of surgery, and there are many cases of deterioration of the results of the operation due to age and related therapeutic pathologies.[2]

Surgery remains the main method of treating chronic stone cholecystitis, especially its complicated types. However, complications after traditional surgical procedures (5-26%) and climate index remain high (0.3-25.5%), especially in patients with concomitant therapeutic diseases that increase the risk of surgery. In patients older than 60 years, it is predicted that the climate index will increase by 2-3 times every next 10 years.

As a result of the experience gained in recent years, the improvement of surgical techniques and equipment, not only the psychology of surgeons, but also the attitude of patients to the operation methods is changing, that is, the desire to get rid of all their diseases at the same time is increasing.[3]

Regarding the need to improve the types of surgical treatment of chronic stone cholecystitis in patients with a risk of surgery, it is known from the above data that two or more diseases that require surgical treatment at the same time in the patients encountered, especially in almost the majority of cases, not only simultaneous operations, but also in the patients with common concomitant therapeutic diseases, which hinder the conduct of simple operations, sharply increase the risk of the operation, using new, modern technologies, which cause less damage to the patient's body , carrying out scientific research in modern abdominal surgery in order to apply, improve existing, create new ones and implement operative treatment methods that are low-cost, have high cosmetic results, are convenient, quick and easier for patients to undergo from a mental

[1] Singh K. K. Et Al. Study Of Associationship Between Gall Stone Composition And Bacteriological Spectrum In Chronic Calculous Cholecystitis //International Surgery Journal. – 2019. – Vol. 6. – №. 8. – Pp. 2741-2744

[2] Laparoscopic Surgery For Common Surgical Emergencies: A Population-Based Study//Lam Cm, Yuen Aw, Chik B Et Al.//Surg Endosc. 2005 Jun; 19 (6):774-9. Epub 2005 May 4.

[3] Shingu Y. Et Al. Laparoscopic Subtotal Cholecystectomy For Severe Cholecystitis //Surgical Endoscopy. – 2016. – Vol. 30. – Pp. 526-531.

aspect It is one of the most well-known needs, which is not only theoretical, but also of great practical importance.

I – CHAPTER

CURRENT PROBLEMS OF SIMULTANEOUS LAPAROSCOPIC OPERATIONS IN PATIENTS WITH A HIGH RISK OF OPERATION

1.1. The role of endosurgical technologies in abdominal surgery in patients with a high risk of surgery

Traditional open surgery is a serious injury to the patient's body, especially in simultaneous operations, the level of injury increases due to the incision, mobilization, and removal of organs.

However, the high trauma of surgical operations and the size of the path to the diseased organ left a negative impact on the results of the treatment. Severe pain syndrome observed in postoperative patients, consistently high complication rates, long hospital stays, postoperative wound suppuration, peritonitis, adherent bowel obstruction, thromboembolic complications, gross and gross scars, ligatured fistulas, frequent occurrence of ventral hernias, long rehabilitation period, etc. increased the risk of reoperation of patients. This situation did not satisfy either the surgeons or the patients. Therefore, research was conducted to create less invasive surgical procedures that are free of these disadvantages.

The most promising direction of minimally invasive surgery is laparoscopic surgery [14,36,45,2]. In 1982, the German K. Zemm performed laparoscopic appendectomy for the first time [113]. Since the 1990s, laparoscopic technologies have been used by Russian surgeons. Yu.I. Gallinger performed the first laparoscopic cholecystectomy operation in Russia in 1991.

In Uzbekistan, cholecystectomy using laparoscopic technology was first performed at the Surgical Research Center of the Republic of Uzbekistan in 1994 by Professor A.V. Vahidov. In a very short time, Sh.I. Karimov et al. (1997), A.E. Ataliev et al. (1997), N.F. Krotov (1998), X.A. Akilov (1998), Sh.K. Atajanov (1999), U.B. Berkinov (2000), U.A. Sherbekov (2001), V.L. Kim (2002) and others gained sufficient clinical experience. Many articles of these authors are devoted to highlighting both positive and negative aspects of endosurgical operations. The deceased academician O'.O. Oripov also described the prospects of this direction in his works.

However, while we were familiar with many works on simultaneous laparoscopic operations in periodical literature, we did not find information about who was the first to use these operations.

Thus, by the 90s of the last century, there were almost no fields left that were not penetrated by videoendoscopic surgery.

By this time, almost all types of "pure laparoscopic" operations had been mastered. Obvious advantages of laparoscopic operations became apparent in cases where the size of the injury caused by the incisions to reach the diseased organ was greater than the injury of the main stage of the operation [15,35,37,76,100].

The further development of laparoscopy, a new technology, was not affected by the size of the injury, the size of the operated organ, its mobilization and removal problems. These problems became more obvious when removing a large resected organ from the abdominal cavity. Such a situation has increased the number of cases of switching from laparoscopic surgery to open surgery. When technical difficulties arise, conversion from laparoscopic operations to open operations is not a complication or failure of the operation. Carrying out the main stages of the operation with laparoscopic technologies, surgeons began to use combined methods to remove a large organ and to perform stages that are technically not possible to perform using laparoscopic technologies. Making a small incision at the specified time and place helped to solve this problem and made it possible to expand the scope of operations [1,38,16,46,90].

In 1991, Meigos introduced the term "laparoscopically assisted surgery" into the practice. In this case, some stages of the operation are performed using a laparoscope, while other stages are performed in an open way with a traditional incision. In the early 90s, this term became popular.

In the periodical literature, information about such rapid popularization of laparoscopic operations, information about new operations began to appear.

Articles about laparoscopic appendectomies [20,55,84,133] and analyzes of their complications [3,26,58,131] began to appear. Various methods of laparoscopic hernioplasty have been used to eliminate abdominal wall hernias [78,94,111,130]. Laparoscopic technologies have also rapidly entered the field of gynecology [20,39,110]. A new slogan appeared: "what can be done by hand can be done with laparoscopic technology."

Thus, endovisual technologies have their place in abdominal surgery and are displacing the traditional methods of open surgery. However, it is one of the most important problems to thoroughly study the tactical and technical aspects of the use of these new technologies, the range of indications and contraindications for them, and to conduct scientific research in this regard.

1.2. Role, problems and prospects of simultaneous laparoscopic operations in abdominal surgery

Simultaneous laparoscopic operations are another significant step forward of the principle of minimal invasiveness mentioned above. With the help of laparoscopic technologies, the possibility of performing two or more operations at the same time increases [19,60,83,101].

According to BJSST data, 20-30% of patients have simultaneous diseases of abdominal organs [21,74,82,120].

In 1989, academician M.I. Perelman called simultaneous operations a new programmed direction in surgery.

Surgical removal of several pathologies at the same time has been of interest to surgeons for a long time. By the 70s of the last century, the development of the diagnostic base, the improvement of the stage of preparing patients for surgery, the improvement of anesthesiological and resuscitation services became the basis for the expansion of the scope of instructions for simultaneous operations [61,75,102,126].

In 1976, professors L.I. Khnox and I.H. Feltshiner from Riga defined simultaneous operations and touched on the main issues of diagnosis and treatment of co-occurring pathologies. The main and simultaneous stages of these operations were clarified and classified. That is, they perfected the existing Reifferscheid classification. Operations performed simultaneously on two or more organs of the abdominal cavity for different pathologies unrelated to each other are called simultaneous operations. They proposed to call the main stage of the operation the stage of elimination of the most dangerous pathology, despite the pre-operative diagnoses. 5 groups of instructions were proposed for simultaneous operations: 1. absolute or curative; 2. preventive; 3. prophylactic; 4. diagnostic; 5. mandatory. It should be noted that this was the most perfect classification at that time [40,77,79].

In his original classification, Lohlein gave only absolute and relative indications for simultaneous operations, and it was more suitable for emergency surgery [62,96].

L.V. Potashev and V.M. Sedov divided simultaneous operations into unexpected, estimated and planned operations [4,46,97].

The initial articles on simultaneous operations aroused great interest among specialists. As a result, heated debates about the definition, classification, tactics, indications and contraindications of simultaneous operations took place. Even so, there is still no clarity about the naming and classification of operations, the only perfectly developed operational tactics.

While reviewing the literature, some authors refer to these operations as "simultaneous operations", others as "joint", or "one-way" operations, and still others as "simultaneous joint" operations. and so on.

K. D. Toskin and V. V. Jebrovsky analyzed these terminological confusions and proposed to call such operations "Simultaneous operations", and we also agree with this opinion. According to the authors, the word "joint" corresponds to the pathology that causes more operations. Thus, operations performed due to "combined" pathologies should be called "simultaneous operations". They emphasize that concomitant diseases that affect the conduct and results of operations should be called background diseases.

The definition of simultaneous operations has always changed. N.N. Malinovsky and L.V. Potashev added to the definition proposed by Feltshiner with Khnox and proposed to call simultaneous operations performed on other organs of the abdominal cavity through one or more surgical incisions. They explained that "combined" pathologies are not pathogenetically related to each other as the main sign of simultaneous operation. This is somewhat controversial, because the pathogenetic relationship may not always be evident [66,85,98,103].

O.B. According to Milonov and others, the main stage of simultaneous operations is called the stage of eliminating the pathology that forced the patient to go to the hospital. This concept is correct only when an absolute diagnosis is made in the pre-hospital period. This is possible only in 36.5% of co-occurring pathologies. Gredjev A.F. (1983) and Xnox L.I. agreeing with the opinion that in patients with competing pathologies, the main disease is the pathology that threatens the health and life of the patient the most.

Different opinions about the types of classification criteria indicate the controversy of statistical indicators and their imprecise interpretation. It has been shown that the total occurrence of simultaneous operations can be from 2.5% to 63% in different sources [47,81,99,109,116]. Such a big difference in numbers A.G. Zemlyanoy (1984) connects with different levels of diagnostic activity in the preoperative period.

Opinions are not the same when expressing the age dependence of the problem under consideration. Some authors [22,44,86] say that patients of working age make up the majority, while others [61,112,121] recognize that co-occurring diseases are more common in middle and old age.

Cases where pathologies with two absolute indications meet can cause confusion in determining which stage of simultaneous operations will be the main one.

In order to summarize the above and eliminate the doubts that have arisen, K.D. Toskin, V.V. Jebrovsky and A.A. Zemlyanikin give a new definition of simultaneous operations. That is, two or more independent operations performed at the same time due to various diseases that require operative treatment are called simultaneous operations. From the article of Knox and Feltshiner, the main and additional stages of simultaneous operations and the structure of the main, combined and accompanying diseases are given.

The term "simultaneous operation" is logically correct, and it seems that the main indications for its implementation arise from the pathologies of various organs that occur together. However, various conditions of patients often affect the size and indications of the operation [5,23,41,129].

The surgeon who decides to perform the second operation assumes a great responsibility both mentally and legally. In such cases, the experience and skills of the surgeon are very important. Because the simultaneous stage of the operation can cause dangerous results for the patient's life [71,114,126].

Lohlein D. (1978) and Pichlmayr [24] suggested dividing simultaneous operations by degrees of severity:

Small operations, operations that do not greatly increase the risk of surgery (appendectomy, hernioplasty, small cystectomies, etc.);

Medium-level operations, operations that increase the surgical wound, but do not significantly increase the risk of the operation (cholecystectomy, prostatectomy);

Operations with a high level of operational risk, operations in cases where the risk of surgical injury and surgery is sharply increased, concomitant diseases are observed;

According to the authors, small and medium operations can be easily performed together. It has been mentioned that this combination of operations will now be included in high-risk operations. Two serious operations can be performed at the same time only according to vital instructions.

Based on this classification Fedorov V.D. (1993) recognize that minor operations can be combined with moderate ones, moderate ones with medium ones, and even medium ones with heavy ones. The author said that severe simultaneous operations should be performed only in cases where the functional indicators of the patients are sufficiently compensated, the surgeon has sufficient qualifications, and the anesthesiological and resuscitation service is at a high level. In cases where the operation poses a great risk to the patient's life, it is emphasized that simultaneous operations should be performed only on the basis of vital instructions.

To this day, discussions about the sequence of second-stage operations such as appendectomy and cholecystectomy continue. Depending on the "purity of the operations", the weight of the main stage, different opinions are emerging in determining the sequence of execution of the simultaneous operation stages.

However, in those years, the main obstacle to the development of simultaneous operations was the large size of the operative section and the damage caused to patients. As a result of any simultaneous operation performed in the traditional way, it leads to an increase in the total number of operative sections and injuries required to perform several operation steps.

Complications after simultaneous operations are reported in the literature to be from 1.5% to 40.2% [17,31,59,73]. These complications depend not only on the nature of joint pathology, but also on the nature of simultaneous operations.

Over time, the euphoria of operations using laparoscopic technologies began to decrease. In this regard, V.S. Savelev (1999) said: "The more the operation became easier for the patient, the more complicated and responsible it became for the surgeon." The fact is that less trauma cannot be a guarantee of a reduction in the occurrence of technical errors and complications (either for "open" or "closed" operations) [81,100,122,132].

Even so, the rapid development of laparoscopic surgery was the main factor to eliminate the failures of performing operations with traditional methods.

Initially, information on simultaneous operations performed simultaneously with laparoscopic cholecystectomy began to appear in periodical literature. By the end of the 1990s, information about serious works on simultaneous laparoscopic operations appeared [6,25,42,118].

Yu.V. Bogdanov, based on his experience, divides simultaneous laparoscopic operations into two groups: simultaneous operations performed only with endovisual technologies and simultaneous operations performed by using open methods with laparoscopic technologies. An example of this is abdominal wall hernioplasty with laparoscopic cholecystectomy.

It is possible to eliminate many different regional pathologies of the abdominal organs at the same time only when using laparoscopic technologies.

K.V. Puchkov writes about the simultaneous operation of Treitz's ligament excision, cholecystectomy, duodenolysis, Hill-Barker modification vagotomy, crurorrhaphy and Nissen method fundoplication using laparoscopic technology.

Similar, laparoscopic hernioplasty [63,91,100,122], adhesion separation [7,27,43,64] operations have been reported by many other authors [87,104,123]. According to some authors [30,51,52,105], necessity and rationality play a very important role in correctly solving the issue of transition to laparotomy. However, the failure of one of the laparoscopic equipment during the operation, the occurrence of complications that cannot be corrected by endosurgery can be a direct indication for conversion. When there are many technical difficulties during the operation with endovisual technology, the transition to laparotomy is the most reasonable way. Reducing the number of laparotomy cases is one of the most important factors in preventing intraoperative complications.

Thus, operations performed with laparoscopic technology, traditional cholecystectomy and appendectomy, abdominal cavity resection and tube removal, herniotomy and hernioplasty, various types of organostomies, and some gynecological operations began to be gradually pushed out of practice.

The emergence of minimally invasive endovideosurgical technologies has opened up new perspectives in expanding the range of indications for simultaneous operations in two or more organs, anatomically distant organs, and this, in turn, should be solved caused a number of problems.

Simultaneous operations have become more important in modern abdominal surgery [18,28,53,119]. In recent years, interest in these operations has been increasing dramatically. There are several reasons for this. Firstly, the increase in the coni and average age of the population and, at the same time, the increase in the number of patients suffering from 2-3 diseases, and secondly, the improvement of diagnostic methods that allow identifying co-occurring pathologies at the stage of outpatient examination (ultrasound, X-ray contrast, computer tomography, etc.) examination methods) and finally, thirdly, advances in modern anesthesiology and resuscitation led to a reduction in the risk of surgery for patients, a significant expansion of the range of indications for simultaneous operations [32,48,72,90].

In recent years, the medical, social and economic effectiveness of joint operations is gaining importance. It is manifested in a decrease in the cost of medicines for the treatment of patients, a decrease in losses in the field of social insurance [125].

However, a number of surgeons [115,124,132] continue to question the feasibility of simultaneous operations because of the increased number and difficulty of operations.

When surgeons come across a gynecological pathology while inspecting the small pelvis, in most cases they refuse to remove it. Because they cannot always correctly approach the size and stages of the operation [65].

Despite the fact that modern diagnostic methods provide high-level information, additional pathologies to the main disease are often found during surgery [92]. This is because A.G. Zemlyanoi (1984) and A.S. Yermolov et al. (1997) believe that when a pathology is diagnosed in preoperative diagnostic examinations, other examinations are stopped. V.G. Sakhautdinov et al. According to (1989), with the increased number of co-occurring diseases in middle-aged and elderly patients, only 3% of patients undergo simultaneous operations. The fate of the remaining patients remains in a very poor condition, although most of them become regular clients of polyclinics and inpatients. Each repeated operation can cause great difficulties from the technical side because of previous operations. That is why A.G. Zemlyanoy (1984), S.N. Hunafin et al. (1988) and I.D. Prudkov (1989) believe and recommend that the operation of local viscerolysis in such patients is necessary in order not to overlook co-occurring pathology.

Due to the diversity of the conditions of their implementation, no clear decision has been reached on the issue of determining instructions and counter-indications for simultaneous operations.

A.F. According to Chernousov (1998), there can be no contraindications to joint operations in planned surgery.

V.Z. According to Makhovskiy (2002), LBBB occurs mainly in patients aged 41 to 70 years (47.77%).

Information about the nature and amount of complications after simultaneous operations is also different. Usually, their level and number depend not only on the specificity of simultaneous operations, but also on the types of co-occurring diseases [10,11,29]. The analysis of articles [88,89,127] shows that the most difficult period after surgery is observed in elderly patients, postoperative complications in patients over 60 years old make 11.1%, and in young people - 2.7%.

According to other authors, the mortality rate after joint operations can be from 5% to 20% [33,49,67]. According to a number of authors, the mortality rate after the above-mentioned operations does not differ from that of single operations [80,106,107]. However, many fatal outcomes have been observed after simultaneous operations, and this is often caused by the presence of additional concomitant therapeutic diseases that worsen the patient's condition [8,68,93].

The reason for the high mortality rate is the general serious condition of the patient, old age, and urgent simultaneous operations. However, there may not be a direct relationship between the size of the operation, the development of complications, and the death rate [50,54,128].

In addition to economic efficiency, simultaneous operations lead to a reduction in the period of reoccupation of the surgical site, a reduction in the period of the patient's incapacity for work, and the elimination of several diseases that require surgical treatment (S.V. Potashev et al., 1997). Indications for simultaneous operations are somewhat limited by the high risk of surgery and greater tissue damage (N.M. Malinovsky et al., 1983).

Simultaneous operations cause great problems, especially in patients with concomitant diseases, such as chronic anemia, obesity, diseases of the cardiovascular system, and previous abdominal surgery. Because, in these patients, not only the risk of surgery, but also the occurrence of postoperative complications are high [9,5695,108,128].

As a result of simultaneous operations performed with the help of laparoscopic technologies, postoperative hernias, eventration, wound suppuration, hematoma formation, and thromboembolic complications in anatomically distant organs are becoming more and more evident [12,34, 69,70].

The main criterion for the successful treatment of co-occurring diseases of the abdominal organs is the perfection of the diagnostic examination measures aimed at identifying the pathologies of the abdominal cavity.

One of the most urgent and fundamental problems is the issue of simultaneous operations performed on women of reproductive age. As a result of the use of endovisual technologies, it is possible to obtain diagnostic materials (exudate, tissue for biopsy) that are not possible during conventional gynecological examinations, along with a visual examination of the pelvic organs. In addition, additional information about the pathological process (whether or not there are adhesions with surrounding tissues, its localization, size, nature, etc.) is obtained [13,57].

In 120 out of 1000 laparoscopic operations performed by S.S. Stebunov (1998), all stages of simultaneous surgical procedures were performed using endovisual technique.

A.V. Galimov (2002) noted significant disturbances of external breathing and hemodynamic parameters during surgery, despite the low trauma of simultaneous laparoscopic operations, quick activation of patients and other advantages. Therefore, when choosing the right treatment method for co-occurring surgical diseases of the abdominal organs, it is necessary to pay special attention to the preoperative and intraoperative treatment of patients with a high risk of cardiovascular complications. have emphasized that it is necessary.

Thus, the review of the literature shows the need for a new interpretation of the range of operations, the development of precise treatment tactical instructions, and the ways to reduce the surgical risk of visiting these organs in co-occurring pathologies of the abdominal organs.

Until now, the importance, role and basic principles of simultaneous laparoscopic operations have not been fully studied. The division of the operation into stages given by some authors is incomplete and does not cover all aspects of the operation.

There is no intraoperative algorithm that determines the sequence and size of the operation stages, and determines the exact work of the surgical team.

There are no specific indications and contraindications for operations.

The laparoscopic technique of these operations is not clearly and clearly explained.

In short, there is no single surgical concept of simultaneous laparoscopic operations.

That's why laparoscopic simultaneous operations are considered one of the most promising directions in abdominal surgery, but simultaneous removal of several pathologies by laparoscopic method causes some discomfort and hesitation among surgeons. Especially in patients with concomitant therapeutic diseases such as chronic anemia, CKD, obesity, which sharply increase the risk of surgery, the cases of joint pathologies of the abdominal organs put surgeons in a difficult situation. It has been witnessed that the periodical literature does not provide sufficient information on the diagnosis of patients with a high risk of such an operation using laparoscopic technologies, that is, information about the stages of simultaneous operation, their sequence, nature and size. we did.

The occurrence of such a situation is related to the theoretical and practical issues of operations performed using laparoscopic technologies that have not yet been solved. A lot of research needs to be done to find a solution to these problems. This study is a small step towards solving this problem.

II – CHAPTER

MATERIALS AND TESTING METHODS

2.1. General description of clinical material

Our scientific research work was based on the results of treatment of 88 patients with *CSC* and *CDAO* and underwent SLO. These patients were treated in the endosurgery departments of the Khorezm Regional Multidisciplinary Medical Center from 2018 to 2023.

Distribution of patients by age and gender is presented in table 2.1.

2.1 Schedule

Distribution of patients by age and gender

Age	Female		Male	
	number	%	number	%
Up to 19	1	0,59	-	-
20 - 44	51	57,73	4	4,76
45 - 59	19	22,02	2	1,78
60 - 74	9	10,71	2	2,38
Total:	80	91,07	8	8,92

The table shows that 91.07% of the researched patients were women. The number of men was 8 and made up 8.92%. More than 85% of patients were aged between 20 and 60 years, and 11 (13.09%) were older than 60 years.

Information about the meeting of *CSC* and *CDAO* is presented in table 2.2. The table shows that *CSC* was used in 14 (19.05%) patients with abdominal adhesions, 9 (12.86%) patients with chronic appendicitis, 11 (16.21%) patients with anterior abdominal wall hernias, 10 It was observed in 1 (16.67%) patients with ovarian cyst and in 3 (5%) patients with uterine myoma. In 13 (21.67%) patients, it was found that there were indications for *LESS*.

Description of the meeting of *CDAO* with chronic stone cholecystitis

№	Type of pathology		Female		Male	
	asosiy	Simultaneous	Number	%	Number	%
1	CSC	Abdominal adhesion disease	10	16.67	4	2,38
2	CSC	Chronic appendicitis	7	11.67	2	1,19
3	CSC	Abdominal wall hernias	9	15.02	2	1,19
4	CSC	Ovarian cyst	10	16.67	-	-
5	CSC	Uterine fibroids	3	5	-	-
6	CSC	LESS*	13	21.67	-	-
7	Total:		52	86.67	8	4,76

*Explanation. Although *LESS* is not a pathology itself, it is included in the table because it is considered as a simultaneous stage of SLO.

When the anamnesis information about *CSC* infection was collected from the patients, we obtained the following results:

Anamnesis up to 1 year was found in 8 (13.33%) patients, anamnesis up to 3 years in 16 (30.77%) patients, and anamnesis up to 5 years and more in 28 (46.67%) patients.

Information about the conducted SLOs is presented in table 2.3.

It can be seen from the table that the most frequently performed SLO was *LC* and joint separation operation and was performed in 20 (22.72%) cases. *LESS* with *LC* was performed in 13 (14.77%) patients, LTSE in 12 (13.63%) patients, LAE in 9 (10.22%) patients, LH in 11 (12.5%) patients, and LM in 5 (5.68%) patients.

As a result of the introduction of endovisual technology into practice, it became possible to perform three, four and even five pathologies at the same time in abdominal organs, which are almost impossible to perform with traditional methods. During our study, we performed such operations in 29 (32.95%) patients. There were 29 cases where more than 2 operations were performed on one patient at the same time. Of these, 5 operations were performed in 1 case, 4 operations in 3 cases, and 3 operations in 25 cases.

General description of simultaneous laparoscopic operation

№	Type of operation		Number	%
	The main stage	Simultaneous stage		
1	LC	separation of contracts	20	22.72
2	LC	Appendectomy	9	10.22
3	LC	Gernioplasty	11	12.5
4	LC	Cystectomy	12	13.63
5	LC	Myomectomy	5	5.68
6	LC	LESS	13	14.77
7	LC	More than 2 operations	18	20.45
8	Total		88	100

Note - there were cases where more than 2 operations were performed on 1 patient at the same time.

The results of the treatment of the patients were divided into 2 groups.

40 patients who underwent SLO were included in the control group. In this group of patients, there were no concomitant therapeutic diseases that significantly increase the risk of surgery in addition to *CSC* and affect its results.

48 patients who underwent SLO were included in the main group. In this group of patients, in addition to *CSC*, there are concomitant therapeutic diseases that increase the risk of surgery and affect its results (moderate and severe levels of chronic anemia, III-IV levels of obesity, IHD, HD and abdominal cavity a cases such as previous surgery have been observed.

The conducted SLOs were divided according to the severity levels according to the classification proposed by D. Lohlein and Pichlmayr (1978):

1. Small simultaneous operations, operations that do not greatly increase the injury and risk of operation;

2. Medium-level operations, operations that increase the injury of the operation, but do not significantly increase the risk of the operation;

3. Operations with a high level of operational risk, operations in cases where the risk of surgical injury and operation is sharply increased, concomitant diseases are observed.

Out of 40 SLOs performed in control group patients, 18 small and 22 medium simultaneous operations were included.

48 SLOs performed in the main group of patients were included in simultaneous operations with a high operational risk.

Preoperative preparation of all patients consisted of a light meal the day before the operation, evening and morning cleansing enemas, and traditional premedication 30 minutes before the operation.

The patients of the main group followed the advice of the necessary specialists (hematologist, therapist, cardiologist, and anesthesiologist) in the pre-operative period and received all the treatments recommended by them.

During our study, we used several improved versions of SLOs performed in the control and main groups: in the control group, we used more traditional methods, and in the main group, we used a movable L-shaped electrode to separate adhesions with *LC*. When performing LA with *LC*, in all cases, after *LC* was performed in the standard way, we used an improved variant of LA (and in the control group, we used variants 1-4). We used 2 methods of LH in both groups of patients.

LESS was carried out in 5 options together with elimination of the main pathology.

It is worth noting that almost 70% of all patients under our observation during the study were women of reproductive age, and 37 of them asked us to perform IJS laparoscopically after the necessary explanations. Because these women had contraindications to other types of contraception.

During our scientific research, we improved and put into practice 7 new laparoscopic surgery methods.

If we take into account the fact that 90% of the population living in the Lower Arolbay region suffer from chronic anemia, there is no doubt how dangerous it is for this category of patients to perform simultaneous operations with traditional methods. In patients with moderate and severe levels of chronic anemia, not only the specifics of the preparatory stage in the preoperative period (hematologist's consultation, hemotransfusion, etc.), is related to the direct operation, but also to anesthesia, the passage of the postoperative period (healing of the wound , volume of treatment procedures, hemotransfusion, etc.) a number of problems may arise.

All patients with chronic anemia followed the hematologist's recommendations and received blood, blood substitutes, hemopoiesis-improving, vitamin, and iron preparations before surgery.

In the control group, 12 (38.7%) of the total patients had chronic iron deficiency anemia, of which 6 (50.0%) had mild, 4 (33.34%) moderate, and 2 (16.66%) severe anemia. . Although 34 patients had moderate and severe levels of chronic anemia, SLOs were fulfilled (Figure 2.1).

2.1 Fig

Percentages of chronic anemia levels in the main group of patients

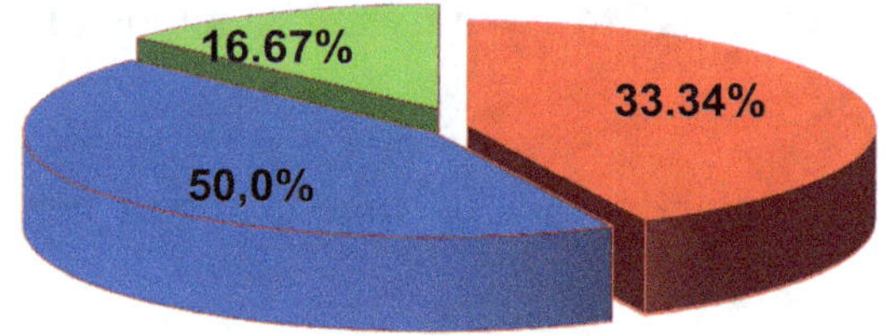

Chronic anemia with iron deficiency was observed in 19 patients (61.29%) in the main group. 9 of these patients (50%) had mild, 6 (33.34%) moderate, and 4 (16.67%) severe chronic anemia. Although 10 patients had moderate and severe levels of chronic anemia, SLOs were fulfilled.

During the study, diseases of the cardiovascular system were observed in 25 (20.45%) of the main group of patients. Among them: 18 (13.63%) patients had HD, 4 (6.81%) patients had IHD (1 patient had a history of myocardial infarction, and 2 patients had a cerebral stroke).

These patients were examined in the pre-operative period after coronary syndrome was eliminated with the help of fast and long-acting nitropreparations according to the recommendations of the cardiologist, the functional condition of the myocardium, ECG, EcoCG, and physical tests were examined and positive changes were detected. It is of great importance that the stage of mentally preparing these patients for the operation is perfect.

In our observations, 14 (15.90%) patients in the main group had III-IV degrees of obesity. Carrying out SLOs in such patients also has its own difficulties. These are: the thickness of the subcutaneous tissue and the front wall of the abdomen, the presence of deep functional and morphological changes in the cardiovascular and respiratory systems.

During our observations, it was found that 8 (16.67%) patients in the main group had previous surgery in their anamnesis. Of these, 2 (4.16%) had acute appendicitis (complicated with diffuse peritonitis), 2 (4.16%) had large anterior abdominal wall hernias, 2 (4.16%) had ovarian cysts, 1 had peptic ulcer disease, and 1 had uterine fibroids. it became known that they conducted an operation on These data and the scars on the anterior abdominal wall were taken into account at the site of abdominal puncture in SLOs.

The following indicators were analyzed in order to assess the tissue damage and the general condition of patients in SLOs:

1. Dimensions of the path to the operated organ (the number of holes in the front wall of the abdomen);

2. Post-operative period (general condition of patients, complaints, results of objective examination, paresis of intestines, length of stay of drainage tubes, etc.);

4. Results of laboratory and instrumental examinations in the postoperative period (USE, X-ray examination, endoscopic examinations, general and biochemical indicators of blood, etc.);

5. The number of anesthesia in the postoperative period;

6. Beginning of patient activation;

7. Number of days;

8. Medicine - consumption of medicine, sewing and bandage materials;

9. The ability of patients to carry out the operation mentally;

10. Cosmetic efficiency.

2.2. General clinical and laboratory instrumental examinations

In order to comprehensively evaluate the general condition of patients, to make a comparative diagnosis of various pathologies, the following examinations were carried out:

1. Clinical examinations: collecting complaints and anamnesis, general examination, palpation of the chest and abdomen, percussion, pulse and control of ABP.

2. Laboratory examination of blood and urine: general analyzes of blood and urine, blood coagulation and coagulogram, bilirubin, determination of transferases, urea, blood sugar, diastase, creatinine, nitrogen metabolism, blood biochemical parameters such as total protein.

3. ECG.

4. Ultrasound examination of the liver and bile ducts, pancreas, spleen, kidneys, lower part of the abdominal cavity, small pelvic organs (on the SSD-630 ultrasound scanner of the Japanese firm "Aloka").

5. EGDFS (with an endoscope CF-10 model of the Japanese company "Olympus").

6. General radiography of the chest and abdomen.

7. Stomach- x-ray examination of the intestinal tract.

8. Gynecologist examination and consultation.

9. Examination and consultation of therapist, anesthesiologist.

All laparoscopic operations were performed under general intubation anesthesia using endosurgical equipment such as "Tantorro" (Germany) and ultrasonic scalpel "Hormonic". The intensity of the light flow was controlled by manual and automatic lighting system devices. We created the pneumoperitoneum with the help of an insufflator with an electronic control system using SO_2 and nitrogen (II) oxide gases. In the second group, in patients with IHD, HD, III-IV degrees of obesity from additional somatic diseases, pneumoperitoneum was created very carefully, in the case of pneumoperitoneum as small as possible (the pressure in the abdominal cavity was reduced by 8-10 mm of wire .without exceeding) SLOs met. An electronic coagulator working in high-frequency "cutting" and "coagulation" mode was used to separate tissues or stop blood. In order to achieve reliable hemostasis during *LC* in patients with severe chronic anemia, ultrasonic coagulation using the URSK - 7N - 22 device was used.

For operations, two laparoscopes (00 and 300), short and long Veresh needles, three trocars of 5 and 10 mm, surgical and anatomical types of "crocodile" clamps, microscissors, dissector, needle holders, spatula and hook-shaped top frequency electrodes, puncture needles, various types of clamps, endo rings, laparoscopic suture apparatus (endo GIA) and other equipment were used.

The use of a combination of equipment and endovisual techniques created the basis for obtaining a stable and high-quality image, as well as the successful implementation of the stages of simultaneous operations.

The complications observed during the study were divided into 3 groups (according to T.B. Duboshina, 1980):

1. Complications related to the performed operations:

a) special (specific)

b) non-specific

2. Complications related to the main pathology.

3. Complications related to concomitant pathology.

The analysis of the received data and statistical processing of numerical indicators was carried out on the "Pentium-IV" computer based on the "Excel" and Access (Microsoft, USA) system programs.

The level of accuracy of the main indicators for groups was determined using the Fisher-Student test. We considered indicators with a difference in the level of compatibility of less than 0.5% ($p < 0.05$) to be accurate.

CHAPTER 3

ANALYSIS OF THE RESULTS OF IMPROVED SIMULTANEOUS LAPAROSCOPIC OPERATIONS IN PATIENTS WITH A HIGH SURGERY RISK, THEIR COMPARATIVE STUDY AND ASSESSMENT OF THEIR ECONOMIC EFFECTIVENESS

3.1. General clinical description of patients

The main group was made up of patients with *CSC* and *CDAO*, suffering from secondary therapeutic diseases that sharply increase the risk of surgery, such as moderate and severe chronic anemia, HD, IHD, III-IV degree obesity, and before surgery on the organs of the abdominal cavity. 88 patients who performed. Distribution of patients by age and gender is given in table 4.1.

4.1 Schedule

Distribution of patients by age and gender

Age	Females		Males	
	number	%	Number	%
Up to 19	-	-	-	-
20-44	40	45,45	2	2,27
45-59	25	28,41	3	3,41
60-74	14	15,91	4	4,54
Total	79	89,77	9	10,23

As can be seen from the table, the majority of patients of this group were women (89.77%). 73.86% of all patients were between 20 and 60 years old, and 15.91% were over 60 years old.

This group was divided according to the type of pathologies identified among the patients as follows: (table 4.2). As it can be seen from the table, *CSC* was more often associated with abdominal adhesion disease (23.86%), ovarian cyst (22.72%), and chronic appendicitis (15.91%). In addition, it was observed in cases of hernias of the anterior abdominal wall (17.04%), uterine fibroids (3.41%). Although *LESS* (17.04%) is not considered a pathology, it is included in this table because it is recognized as a simultaneous stage of SLOs.

Types of pathology identified in the main group of patients

№	Type of pathology		Ayollar		Erkaklar	
	main	Simultaneous	soni	%	soni	%
1	CSC	Abdominal adhesion disease	16	18,18	5	5,68
2	CSC	Chronic appendicitis	12	13,63	2	2,27
3	CSC	Abdominal wall hernias	12	13,64	3	3,41
4	CSC	Ovarian cyst	20	22,72	-	-
5	CSC	Uterine myoma	3	3,41	-	-
6	CSC	LESS	15	17,04	-	-
7	Total		78	88,64	10	11,36

*Explanation. Although LESS is not a pathology itself, it is included in the table because it is considered as a simultaneous stage of SLO.

The anamnesis of *CSC* disease was as follows:

20 (22.72%) patients had an anamnesis up to 1 year, 34 (38.63%) up to 3 years, and more than 5 years in 34 (38.63%) patients.

Operations performed on patients of this group are presented in table 4.3.

Types of operations performed in the main group of patients

№	Type of operation		Number	%
	Main stage	Simultaneous		
1	LC	Separation of contracts	8	16.67
2	LC	Appendectomy	6	12.50
3	LC	Hernioplasty	7	14.58
4	LC	Cystectomy	9	18.75
5	LC	Myomectomy	3	6.25
6	LC	LESS	7	14.58
7	LC	More than 2 operations	8	16.67
8	Total		48	100

Note - there were cases where more than 2 operations were performed on 1 patient at the same time.

As can be seen from the table, the most performed SLOs are *LC* and adhesion separation (16.67%), *LC* and ovarian cyst removal (6.25%), *LC* and LA 12.50%, *LC* and LH 14.58%, *LC* and *LESS* was performed in 14.58%, *LC* and LM in 6.25% of patients. There were 8 cases where more than 2 operations were performed on one patient at the same time. Of these, 2 operations were performed in 1 case, 2 operations in 1 case, and 1 operation in 7 cases.

All SLOs performed in this group of patients were included in severe simultaneous operations according to the classification proposed by D. Lohlein and Pichlmayr (1978).

All operations performed on patients of this group were performed under general intubation anesthesia. In the period of preoperative preparation, the patients were instructed to eat a light meal the day before the operation, and a cleansing enema was administered in the evening and on the morning of the operation. 30 minutes before the operation, he was premedicated as usual.

Table 4.4 shows the average time spent on SLOs conducted in the main group of patients. It is clear from the table that the longest time is *LC* and LSE, 106.40±1.52 minutes to separate contracts, 97.21±2.05 minutes to *LC* and LA, 93 to transfer *LC* and LH, It took 73±2.15 minutes. The least time was 54.40±1.40 minutes for *LC* and *LESS*, and 71.10±1.12 minutes for *LC* and LC.

4.4 Schedule

Average duration of SLOs in the main group (minutes)

Main stage	Simultan stage	The average duration of the operation (minute)
LC	Separation of contracts	79,42±1,35
LC	LESS	54,40±1,40
LC	*LC*	71,10±1,12
LC	*LA*	97,21±2,05
LC	*LH*	93,73±2,15
LC	Myomectomy	76,33±0,33
LC	*LC*, LESS	79,40±1,76
LC	LC, Separation of contracts	106,40±1,52

As usual, the majority of patients hospitalized with CSC were women. It was found that ovarian cysts, uterine fibroids, secondary infertility, and similar pathologies are more common among these patients. It is known that the removal of pathologies of small pelvic organs with cholecystectomy in such patients by traditional methods is difficult for the surgeon and a serious injury for the patient. Solving these problems can be achieved only as a result of the use of endovisual technologies, which have very high possibilities.

Of the 88 patients observed in the main group, 36 (40.90%) were admitted to the hospital with co-occurring pathology requiring surgery, and 16 (18.18%) patients had a third additional pathology in direct inpatient examinations. determined as a result. Intraoperative pathology presents a very difficult problem for the surgeon. What to do? Should we limit ourselves to an operation that eliminates the pathology that caused the patient to go to the hospital, or should we also eliminate the pathology that was found? What should be the tactics, scope, character of the operation? It is required to find the optimal answer to such questions in a short time. Because there was no preoperative preparation stage and plan to eliminate the found pathology.

4.5 Schedule

Description of additional pathologies found during the intraoperative period

Pathology name	Number	%	Males		Females	
			number	%	number	%
Adhesion disease	10	38,46	1	3,84	9	34,61
Ovarian cyst	12	46,15	-	-	12	46,15
Chronic appendicitis	2	7,69	-	-	2	7,69
Uterine myoma	2	7,69	-	-	2	7,69
Total	26	100	1	3,84	25	96,15

In the course of our study, we conducted SLO in the same patients and came to the conclusion that it should be performed in all cases where there are opportunities to eliminate the pathology found during the intraoperative period. The description of the conducted SLOs is given in table 4.5.

One of the main factors preventing the large-scale implementation of SLOs is their legal and organizational aspects. For example, in the case of gynecological diseases that occur together with gallstones, the involvement of a gynecologist in the operating team is the basis for preventing tactical mistakes, choosing the size and nature of the operation correctly, and conducting it optimally.

During the research, after gaining certain experience, we performed operations to eliminate uterine fibroids, ovarian cysts and similar gynecological pathologies together with specialist gynecologists.

3.2. Abdominal operations performed with simultaneous laparoscopic cholecystectomy

In all cases, the main phase of SLOs, which were also performed in the main group, was organized by *LC*. In 20 (23.86%) cases, the main pathology was observed together with abdominal adhesion disease. Because this condition is often located around the gallbladder, scrotal tumor, ovaries, and other organs, patients with *CSC*, on inquiry, in addition to right subcostal pain, gastrointestinal discomfort, that is, nausea, vomiting, flatulence, flatulence and other similar complaints were observed. It was found that these complaints were formed due to the adhesion of the transverse colon, duodenum, stomach and other organs to the adhesion process around the gallbladder.

In 6 (6.81%) patients, the bulbous part of the duodenum and the pyloric canal, the large intestine were attached to the Hartmann's pouch of the gall bladder, and in 3 patients, the rest of the stomach and the duodenum, the hepatoduodenal ligament were completely attached to this area. it was found that the big car that he had closed was stuck. In order to prevent iatrogenic damage to the pyloric canal and duodenum, it was necessary to separate adhesions not only from the gallbladder wall, but also from its serous layer.

Carrying out SLOs in patients who have previously undergone surgery on the organs of the abdominal cavity has gained special importance and caused specific difficulties. This is especially observed when there is a postoperative scar on the white line of the abdomen near the navel. It was found that 15 (17.04%) patients had previous surgery in their anamnesis. Of these, 6 (6.81%) had acute appendicitis (complicated with diffuse peritonitis), 3 (3.41%) had large anterior abdominal wall hernias, 4 (45.45%) had ovarian cysts, and 1 had gastric ulcer disease. , 1 was found to have undergone an operation for uterine myoma. In such patients, it is very important to enter the Veresh needle and the first trocar into the abdominal cavity. Because there is a high risk of uncontrolled insufflation of gas into the abdominal cavity and injury to the hollow organs. In our opinion, it would be correct to determine the most convenient point for puncture and the first trocar in these patients from the left flank area, because adhesion process was observed the least after previous open operations in this area. The remaining points are made from the most convenient areas under the control of a laparoscope (Fig. 4.1).

4.1 Figure

Insertion points of trocars on the anterior abdominal wall in patients who have undergone previous surgery

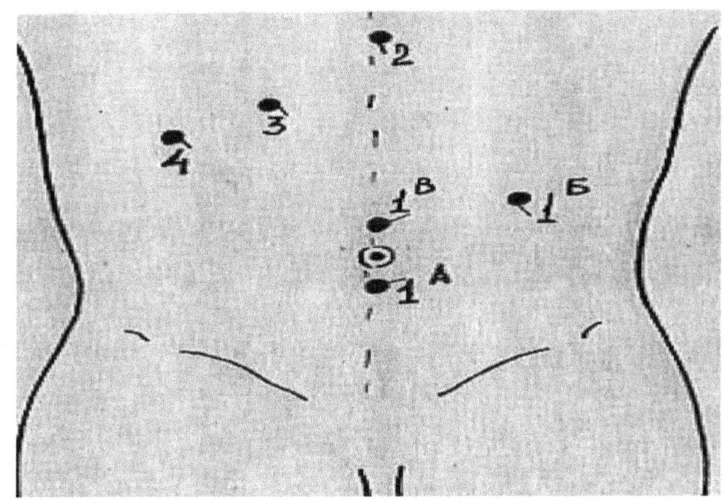

1a. For Veresh needle and 1st trocar. 1b. The second option for the 1st trocar. 2. For a second trocar of 10 mm. 3 - 4. For trocars with 5 mm.

We selected the first point for creating a pneumoperitoneum and serving as a port for the laparoscope individually for each patient. It was taken into account the degree of development of the subcutaneous tissue, the previous operation, and the presence of signs of intestinal obstruction due to adhesions. Since 18 (35,23) patients did not have umbilical hernia or postoperative scars in this area, we chose point 1a below the navel as the first point. In patients with umbilical hernia or postoperative scars below the umbilicus along the white line of the abdomen (5.7 and 2.8%), we used point 1b above the umbilicus to enter with a trocar.

This point was also used in patients with IV degree obesity. After inserting a laparoscope into the abdominal cavity from the first point, the abdominal cavity was examined in detail. Further tactics depended on the results of the inspection. If adhesions were found in the subhepatic and hepatoduodenal areas, the second manipulator was inserted into the abdominal cavity from the right flank (8 cases). Entered from the area under a (in 3 cases). As a result of the location of the attachment process on the upper floor of the abdominal cavity, we had to use the second manipulator in 3 cases to the left of the navel, from the lateral edge of the rectus muscle, and in 7 cases to the same point on the right side. Usually, manipulators inserted from two 5-mm trocars are sufficient to separate adhesions, but in 5 cases it was necessary to insert 3 x 5-mm trocars. After the formation of pneumoperitoneum, adhesions formed between large intestine, intestines and anterior abdominal wall become visible and easy to separate. In 11 of 21 such patients, it was found that the anterior abdominal wall, large intestine, transverse colon and liver were involved in the adhesion process. In cases of obesity of the IV degree and a lot of fatty tissue in the round neck of the liver (6.38%), we introduced the main manipulator from point 2b. A 10-mm trocar is inserted through the lateral edge of the round liver, making it easier to work in the subhepatic area.

Therefore, it is advisable to plan all the procedures to be performed in advance and use the holes made in the front wall of the abdomen.

Separation of contracts using the above-mentioned methods has its own disadvantages. For example, it takes a lot of time to separate adhesions, the reliability of hemostasis is not high. Therefore, we used these methods only at the beginning of our research. Later, we created a "mobile" L-shaped electrode that facilitates the cutting of adhesions in the abdominal cavity and used it in 21 patients. In cases of advanced adhesions, as a result of the use of a "mobile" L-shaped electrode, the time of separation of adhesions is reduced several times, reliable hemostasis is achieved and separation of adhesions is easier, because in this case adhesions are "collected" and brought to a state of compression and cut in place, tearing of the serous layer of the intestine (deserosis), complications such as bleeding are not observed (Figure 4.2).

4.2 Figure

Adhesion separation using a movable L-shaped electrode

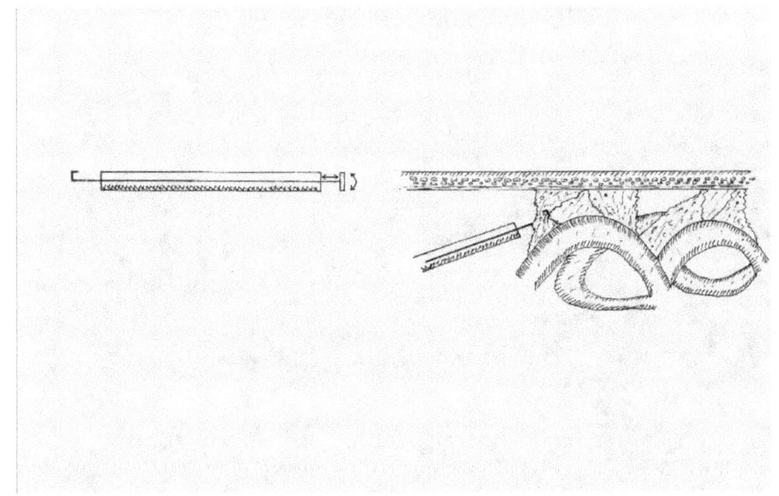

Usually, we start *LC* as far from the choledox as possible, in the neck of the gallbladder. After identification of the bile duct of the gallbladder, it is clipped. In cases where the standard clip does not fit the gallbladder artery (in its band type) (in 7 patients), it is separated from the maximally close places to the gallbladder with a coagulator using an L-shaped electrode. After the gallbladder is removed, if there are signs of bleeding from its place, coagulation is performed with the help of clamp or shovel-shaped electrodes.

During our study, skin incisions, intra-abdominal insertion of trocars, tissue dissection, gallbladder artery and bile duct clipping, gallbladder dissection and replacement were performed. we developed a new method. This method consists in cutting the skin with an ultrasound knife with a low-frequency resonant vibration frequency of 23.9-26.9 kHz, a power of 0.2-0.4 W/cm2 and a current of 6-8 mA (invention received a preliminary patent from the State Patent Office, IDP 04858). An ultrasonic scalpel with a length of 20-50 cm and a diameter of 5-10 mm, equipped with a special waveguide, is inserted into the abdominal cavity through the epigastric port, and the gallbladder is treated with it. Point ultrasound coagulation is continued from top to bottom until a thin but solid film is formed (Figure 4.3).

4.3 Figure

Ultrasonic device URSK-7N-22

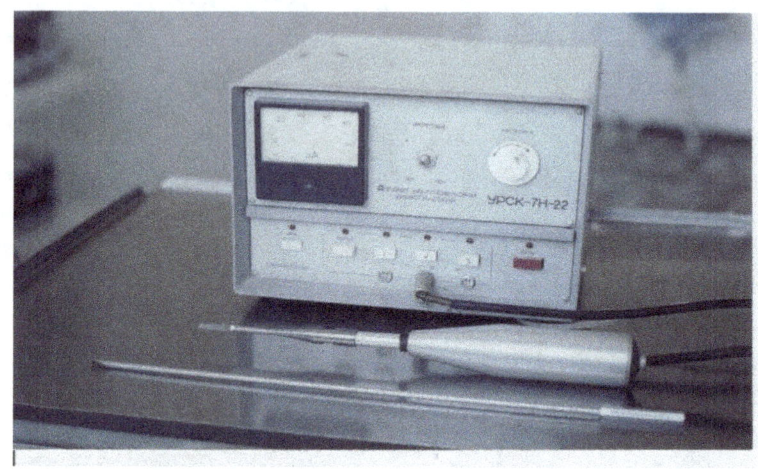

The frequency of ultrasound vibrations is 26.6 kHz, the duration of the treatment for the gallbladder should be up to 10-15 minutes. In this way, *LC* was performed in 17 (19.32%) patients.

Thus, the method we proposed for dissection of adhesions with *LC* in patients with *CSC* disease and previous abdominal surgery, that is, dissection of adhesions using a movable L-shaped electrode, is a quick, easy procedure for this stage of the operation. , thorough and, most importantly, reliable hemostasis was achieved.

Simultaneous laparoscopic cholecystectomy and appendectomy

CSC and chronic appendicitis were found together in 9 (10.22%) cases. When the complaints and anamnesis of patients with this *CSC* were analyzed in depth and purposefully, it was noted that in addition to the typical anamnesis and complaints of this disease, they also have pains in the right flank area that appear from time to time, often of a radiating nature. . Chronic appendicitis is suspected in patients with such complaints. Because these patients were informed about the possibilities of laparoscopic technologies, they also agreed to LA operation together with *LC*. In these patients, during diagnostic laparoscopy, there are adhesions in the area of the vermiform tumor and signs of chronic inflammation of the tumor (deformation, uneven thickening of the walls of the vermiform tumor, focal hypertrophy, signs of atrophy, etc.) is planned to be held.

The technique of performing simultaneous *LC* and LA was as follows: 1 and 2 x 10 mm trocars and 3 x 5 mm trocars were inserted from the standard points while inserting the trocars into the abdominal cavity for *LC* surgery, taking into account the LA stage. if inserted, a 10-mm trocar was inserted instead of the 4th 5-mm trocar from the Mc Burney point in the right flank area. Other stages of *LC* were performed in the usual conventional manner. Then the laparoscope was moved to the port in the epigastric region. Then, an additional 5 mm trocar was inserted from the left side, and the patient's position was changed to that of the LTSE operation, and the right side was raised to 15-200. We used several traditional variants of LA in the initial stages of our study and in control group patients. These methods have been used more and more to perform single LAs, allowing to select the most convenient options as a stage of SLO and to be performed not only together with *LC*, but also with other laparoscopic operations (LTSE, LH, separation of adhesions). . We used *LC* and LA together in several options, improving the methods used in control group patients and eliminating their shortcomings.

The first option. During our study, we tested another new method of LAas a stage of SLO (in 2 cases). Its performance is as follows: after the *LC* stage of SLO is performed, the laparoscope is transferred to the epigastric port and under its control, a 10 mm trocar is inserted from the right flank area. The apical part of the tumor was held up with clamps, then a bipolar electrode was inserted from the port in the umbilical region and separated from the tumor handle through the serous layer by means of bipolar coagulation. With this, reliable hemostasis was achieved. Then, two endorings were introduced, the first one was passed from the base of the tumor, and the second one was connected 1 cm above the first one, and it was cut with bipolar coagulation 6-7 cm above the first connected ring using a bipolar electrode. The tumor pocket was thermally treated with bipolar coagulation. The tumor was removed from the port in the right flank area (an application for the invention was submitted to the State Patent Office, IAP 20030843). But the advantages of this method over the options listed above were not what we expected.

The second option. A 10-mm trocar in the right flank region of the worm-like tumor is grasped with clamps from the terminal part and taken out together with the dome from the port in the right flank region expanded with an expander. Appendectomy is performed in an extracorporeal way in a simple way, and the cyst of the worm-like tumor is inserted into the dome of the cecum with the help of a cystic suture and peritonized with a Z-shaped suture. After that, the dome of the caecum is lowered into the abdominal cavity (Figure 4.4). In our opinion, this option of LA is the most ideal option, whether it is performed separately or as a simultaneous operation. But this option can be used in cases where the thickness of the abdominal wall is not more than 4-5 cm, the dome of the cecum is mobile and there are no adhesions with the surrounding tissues, and during our research, this method was used in 3 patients. LA conducted.

4.4 Figure

Extracorporeal laparoscopic appendectomy

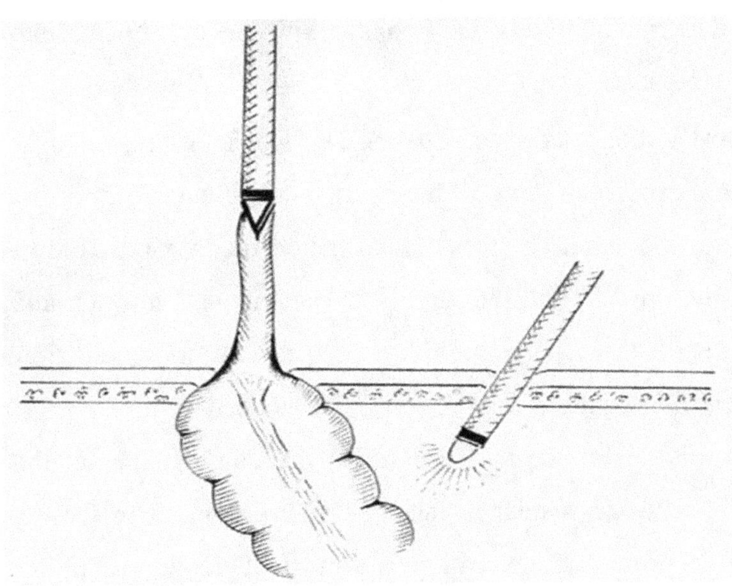

The above-mentioned known and created by us and other (typical, rings, clips, GIA, coagulation, US LAs, etc.) variants of LA are not without a number of shortcomings. Either they are carried out individually (not as a simultaneous operation) or as a simultaneous operation. The main reason for this is the relative complexity of the cystic and Z-shaped sutures, which is the essential and important stage of appendectomy, and the cystic tumor sac is buried in the cecal dome.

Other stages of appendectomy: separation of adhesions, suturing, ligation, separation, ligation and cutting of the appendix are performed using special laparoscopic equipment (endo GIA, rings, bipolar coagulation, US). easy, fast and reliable. Therefore, proponents of LA believe that there is no need to sink the helminthic cyst into the cecal dome in LA and complete LA without sinking the appendix cyst into the cecal dome. In such cases, information and facts about the complications associated with this stage are almost not given in the periodical literature (that is, negative cases are not recorded), so the results are considered positive.

Taking into account all of the above and taking into account the need to sink the scrotum into the cecal dome in any type of appendectomy, especially if it is a simultaneous operation, we recommend the newly improved method of LA (i.e. we have created a helminthic tumor sac (which allows the cyst to sink into the dome of the cecum in almost all cases).

The third option. As a stage of SLOs, we have created a new improved method of LA, which maintains all the positive advantages of the above options of LA and negates the negative sides. This method made it possible to perform the operation easily, quickly and thoroughly in patients with a thick abdominal wall, that is, obese patients, in patients with a deep cecum dome and limited mobility. The essence of this method is as follows: 2 P-shaped sutures passing through all layers of the anterior abdominal wall from the edge of the wound are slightly expanded with a port expander at the Mack-Burney point in the right flank area (from the projection of the vermiform tumor). Threads are tightly pulled and connected, thereby achieving maximum (up to 5-10 times) thinning of the front wall of the abdomen.

With the help of these threads, the abdominal wall can be moved in the desired direction - up, down, right and left, and deepened into the abdominal cavity. Then, the apical tumor is grasped with forceps and pulled out of the abdominal cavity together with a part of the dome of the cecum. Even if the movement of the cecal dome is limited, as a result of the application of these P-shaped sutures, which compress the abdominal wall, in almost all cases (100% in our observations), the stage of appendectomy outside the abdominal cavity can be performed in the traditional way, with simple equipment. To do this, it is possible to anchor the tumor pocket to the cecal dome with the help of a kisset and Z-shaped (if necessary) sutures. In this way, LA was performed in 9 patients (Figure 4.5).

4.5 Figure

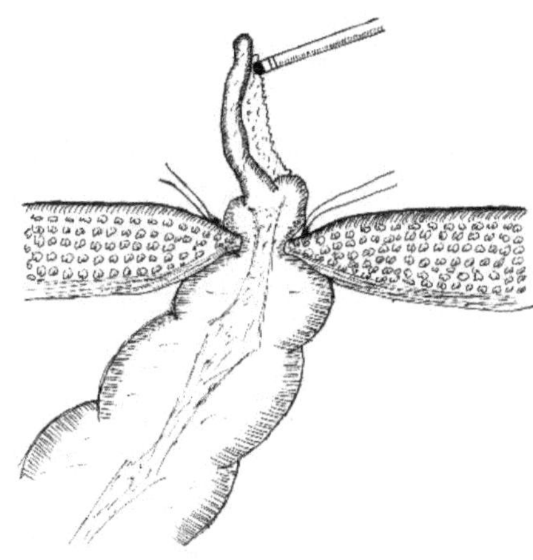

As a result of using this method, there were no technical difficulties or unexpected adverse events. This method made it possible to perform LA accurately, carefully, and reliably even in obese patients. The use of this method in cases where the helminthic tumor is located retrocecally or retroperitoneally can make the operation technique (traditional and LA) much easier.

Thus, LA performed as a simultaneous step to *LC* (in 14 patients) is the most convenient of the above-mentioned methods and the last is its improved third method.

Abdominal white line and umbilical hernias were observed in 15 (17.04%) patients together with *CSC*, and the size of the hernia gate was greater than 4 cm. LH was performed together with *LC* in these patients. The hernia gate was closed with a special polypropylene mesh and eliminated. The execution technique is as follows: The skin and subcutaneous tissue over the hernia is cut longitudinally or transversely by 1.5-2 cm. When the hernia sac was found, it was opened and the organ inside was determined to be viable, then it was inserted into the abdominal cavity. Then a 10 mm trocar was inserted into the abdominal cavity from this place and sealed with 2-4 stitches. The *LC* phase of the SLO was performed in the usual way. Then, a pre-prepared polypropylene mesh was inserted into the abdominal cavity from the trocar in the epigastric area to close the hernial gate (when the hernial gate is larger than 4 cm). The size of the mesh should be 2-4 cm wide and 2 cm longer than the size of the hernial gate (after straightening). On the edges of the net, there are 8 to 12 lavsan threads, 15-20 cm long, which are easy to pull out with a hook needle. The distance between the threads should not be greater than 15-20 mm. To prevent the threads from getting tangled, the edge of the net was tied with thin kapron threads. After being inserted into the abdominal cavity, the mesh was straightened and brought to the area of the hernial gate with a clamp. Then, the lavsan threads on the edge of the mesh were pulled under the skin with the help of a hooked needle. In this case, the needle should enter the abdominal cavity 2 cm away from the edge of the hernial gate. After pulling out all the threads, they were tied under the skin (over the aponeurosis). With this method, the polypropylene mesh was attached to the hernial gate without too much tension and the hernial gate was eliminated. All the manipulations listed above were performed under strict laparoscope control (Fig. 4.6).

4.6 Figure

Hernioplasty using polypropylene mesh

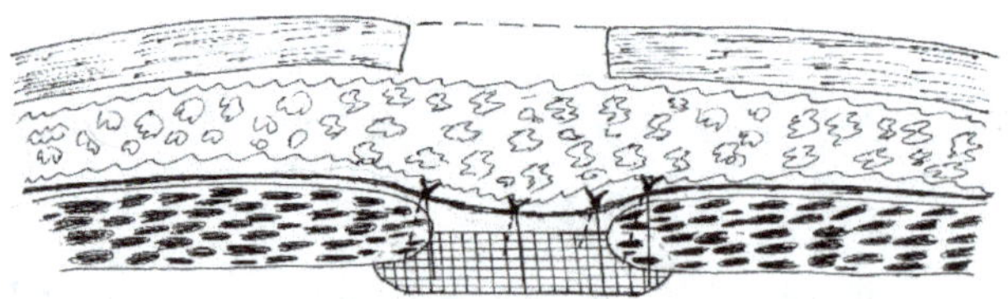

As a result of the application of the above-mentioned LGP method, the foundation was created for the solid, non-pulling closing of the Churra gate, and for quick, accurate and thorough operation under visual control.

Laparoscopic cholecystectomy and cystectomy

Since the majority of *CSC* patients are women, it was necessary to pay special attention to their gynecological conditions during preoperative examinations. Cystectomy surgery was performed laparoscopically in all patients (12 patients) who were diagnosed with an ovarian cyst with *LC*. Patients were examined by a gynecologist in the pre-operative period and an indication for cystectomy was determined. In these patients, we performed the *LC* stage of SLO in the order indicated above. When choosing the points for trocars, the side of the cyst, the body structure of the patients, and previous surgery were taken into account. After performing the *LC* stage of SLO, the position of the patient on the operating table was changed, i.e., the head side was raised 20 - 250 degrees down, the leg side was raised 25 - 300 degrees. Depending on the size, character, and location of the cyst (on the leg, adherent, intraligamentary, etc.), the LTSE stage of SLO was performed as follows.

As a result of our use of LTSEs of the above variants in the elimination of ovarian cysts in the early stages of our study and in patients of the control group, it became clear that these variants are not without their own shortcomings. That is, despite the fact that in the first option presented in chapter 3, less time is spent on removing the cyst, and it is a less traumatic and organ-preserving operation method, the probability of cyst re-formation (recurrence) is higher. taking into account that it takes more time and is technically more complicated, and the fourth option was difficult to perform in patients with III-IV obesity, we used the improved option of LTSE. After the *LC* stage of SLO, regardless of the size of the ovarian cyst, it was punctured under the control of a laparoscope and the liquid inside was aspired. Then the laparoscope was moved from the paraumbilical port to the epigastric port.

A 10 mm trocar was inserted into the abdominal cavity in the suprapubic region. Then, the anterior abdominal wall is deepened, and in almost all cases, P-shaped sutures passing through all layers of the abdominal wall are placed from both ends of the trocar to create conditions for extracorporeal cystectomy and make it more convenient. These stitches are tied tightly. As a result, the abdominal wall thinned several times. With the help of these threads, it was possible to move or sink the abdominal wall in the desired direction - up, down, right and left. Then, one end of the cyst wall was clamped and taken out of the abdominal cavity with a foot. The base of the cyst leg was sutured in the usual manner and the cyst was excised. The bag was inserted into the abdominal cavity (extracorporeal cystectomy, Fig. 4.7).

4.7 Figure

Extracorporeal cystectomy with P-shaped suture

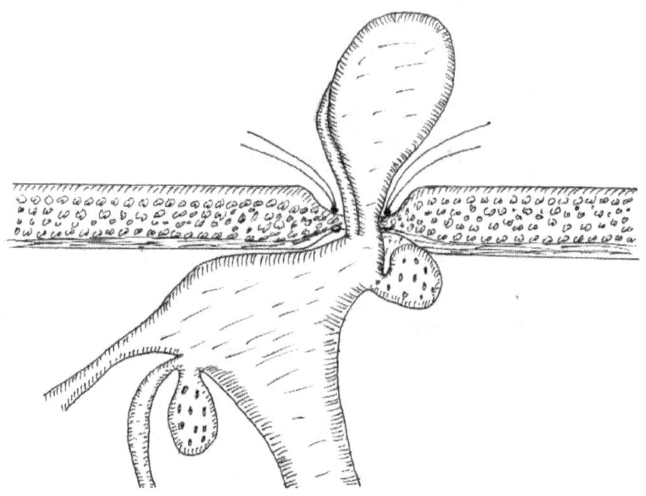

As a result, it was possible to perform this stage of SLO reliably, accurately, quickly and easily. The main condition for performing this stage of SLO is that regardless of the size of the cyst, the cyst should be in the leg and it should be mobile. During our research, we are convinced that this method is more effective and reliable than other methods, and we have recently used this method in up to 95% of cases (20 cases). The possibility of using this method is limited when the cyst forms adhesions with the surrounding tissues and its mobility is limited, when it is intraligamentary.

Thus, it is appropriate to perform simultaneous operations with the use of the improved method of LTSE in patients with III-IV degree of obesity, who have an ovarian cyst together with *CSC*.

Laparoscopic cholecystectomy and elective surgical sterilization

In 13 patients (17.04%) who were infected with *CSC* and had indications for *LESS*, *LESS* operation with *LC* was performed. *LESS* was guided by women's wishes and the presence of contraindications to other types of contraception. Taking into account that the *LESS* stage of the simultaneous operation can be easily performed from the trocar insertion points required for the *LC* stage, the first trocar was inserted as usual from the paraumbilical area. In women with normosthenic and asthenic body structure (9), 2nd, 3rd, 4th trocars were inserted into the abdominal cavity, taking into account the planned *LC* and *LESS*. That is, the 2nd trocar was inserted from the epigastric area, the 3rd trocar was inserted from the right subcostal area, and the 4th trocar was inserted from the right flank area. In patients with III-IV degree of obesity (6), one of the 5-mm trocars had to be inserted slightly lower than in the previous cases, and in 4 cases, the analog trocar had to be inserted from the left iliac region. . After completing the main steps of *LC*, we transferred the laparoscope from the parumbilical port to the epigastric port and changed the position of the patient on the operating table. That is, if we raised the lower part of the body by 30-400, we lowered the head. This situation led to the displacement of the intestines and large intestine to the upper parts of the abdominal cavity and improved visibility in the pelvic cavity. Once the fallopian tubes were identified, their occlusion was performed in the following manner. In contrast to the 4 methods presented in the above chapter, this method is much easier, faster and more reliable in terms of execution technique, in which the position of the patient on the operating table is changed after the *LC* stage of SLO is performed. Then, a segment of the fallopian tube was cut from the place closest to the uterus by coagulation using a bipolar coagulator (in 11 cases) (Figure 4.8).

LESS performed with the removal of one segment using bipolar coagulation.

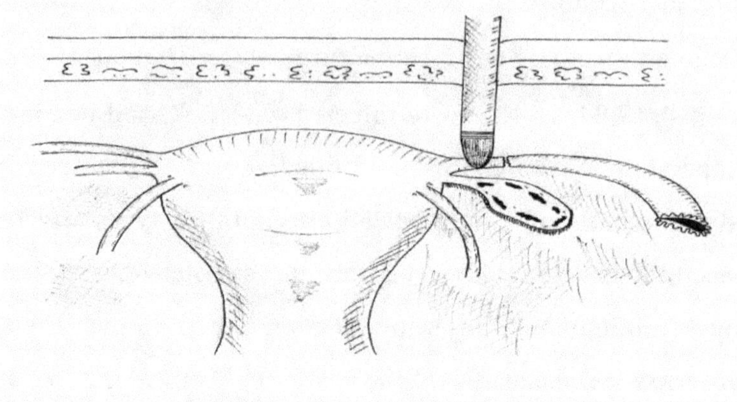

Therefore, taking into account the above, it is worth noting that the joint implementation of HEC and *LESS* by laparoscopic method is an easy, convenient, accurate operation that saves women not only from chronic stone cholecystitis, but also from uncomfortable and dangerous relieves the use of contraceptive methods. The *LESS* methods listed above are more reliable, faster, and more accurate than others.

Although performing *LESS* in combination with *LC* has been done in many variants, it seems that the scientific novelty is not very well represented. However, it should be noted that with the help of laparoscopic technologies, there is an excellent opportunity to perform 3, 4 or even more operations at the same time, which indicates the high practical importance of this department.

Laparoscopic cholecystectomy and myomectomy

Simultaneous *LC* and myomectomy was performed in 5 (5.68%) patients. In these patients, it was found that the myomatous nodes were located in the subserosal area and their size was not larger than 9 weeks, and they were an indication for laparoscopic myomectomy. After *LC*, which is the main stage of SLO, we changed the position of the patient on the operating table to that of LTSE. An additional 10-mm trocar was inserted into the abdominal cavity from the left side. Then, with the help of bipolar coagulation, we separated the myomatous node from the surrounding tissues (Figure 4.9).

4.9 Figure

Removal of myomatous node using bipolar coagulation

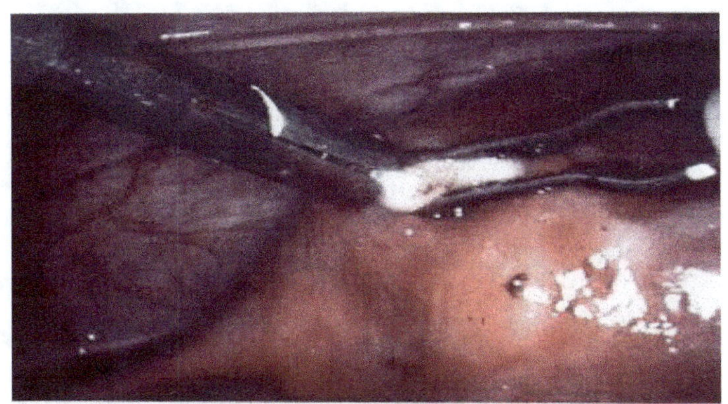

Thus, our experiences indicate that in cases where *CSC* and uterine fibroids occur together or in cases where a myomatous node is an intraoperative finding, it is a convenient opportunity to perform myomectomy together with *LC*.

It is known that the organs of the abdominal cavity, which are anatomically far away from each other, can detect simultaneous pathologies at the same time, with less damage to the patient, less cost, and a precise, thorough, correct sequence of operation steps. It is very difficult to eliminate using traditional methods. However, in such cases, these problems can be solved by using laparoscopic technology. From the information presented above, it is known and clear that it is possible to perform not two or three, or even five operations on one patient at a time without any risk to the patient, only after carrying out the necessary procedures in the pre-operative period. , the following example confirms that it can be performed with the help of laparoscopic technologies.

It is known that in patients suffering from concomitant somatic diseases such as diseases of the cardiovascular system, chronic anemia, obesity, etc., it is almost impossible to safely perform not one but 4 operations at the same time with traditional methods. there is no way. Our above example confirms that such operations can be performed safely and accurately at the same time only with the help of laparoscopic technologies, only after carrying out the necessary procedures in the pre-operative period.

3.3. Simultaneous laparoscopic operations in patients with a high risk of surgery

One of the main factors preventing the desired surgical treatment, especially operations on the abdominal organs, is the patient's (apart from surgical pathologies) and today's common concomitant therapeutic diseases. Chronic anemia ranks first among these diseases. That is why this category of patients is still at a high risk of performing simultaneous operations at *CDAO*. Especially, such a situation is clearly reflected in the joint surgical elimination of pathologies of the pelvic cavity organs, which are infected with *CSC* disease. In order to eliminate such simultaneous pathologies through existing traditional open methods, it is necessary to expand the upper middle laparotomy incision or to make a separate incision for cholecystectomy, to eliminate pelvic cavity pathology. As a result of this, it is natural to lose a lot of blood, in simple uncomplicated cholecystectomy or appendectomy operations, blood loss ranges from 100 ml to 500 ml, while in simultaneous operations, this figure is at least twice as much.

If we take into account the occurrence of chronic anemia in 90% of the population living in the lower Arolbay region, an ecologically unfavorable region, there is no doubt how dangerous it is for patients to perform simultaneous operations with traditional methods. In patients with moderate and severe levels of chronic anemia, it is not only related to the specificity of the preparatory stage in the preoperative period (hematologist's consultation, hemotransfusion, etc.), but also directly related to the operation, narcosis, and the postoperative period (healing of the wound, volume of treatment procedures, hemotransfusion, etc.) a number of problems may arise. Therefore, the importance of laparoscopic, especially SLO, increases dramatically in this category of patients. Both theoretically and practically, it is an indisputable fact that the negative impact of laparoscopic injury on the body and the amount of blood loss are extremely low compared to traditional operations. However, we did not find any specific facts about the experience of using SLOs in this category of patients in the periodical literature. That is, they did not pay enough attention to this important situation. But it is clear that the amount of blood lost during surgery in patients with chronic anemia is much higher than in patients without anemia. Because, as we mentioned above, hemostatic properties of blood are severely disturbed in patients with chronic anemia. According to our calculations, blood loss in normal conventional (typical, uncomplicated) *LC* or LAE was 30-60 ml in patients without chronic anemia, and in patients with chronic anemia and it was 50-90 ml. It is natural that this indicator is much higher in SLOs, especially in complex and complicated operations.

Taking into account the above, the importance of laparoscopic, especially SLO, increases in patients with chronic anemia. For this reason, we performed the following technique of SLOs in patients with chronic anemia: to introduce trocars, only the epidermis layer of the skin wound was cut with a scalpel, and the next dermis layer was cut using a fine needle electrode. When inserting trocars of 10 and 5 mm, lesviated conical, pyramidal conical, blunt yescentric (ZEROCART), trocars of conical shape with slightly blunted tips were used (Figure 4.10).

4.10 Figure

Trocars used in SLOs performed in patients with chronic anemia

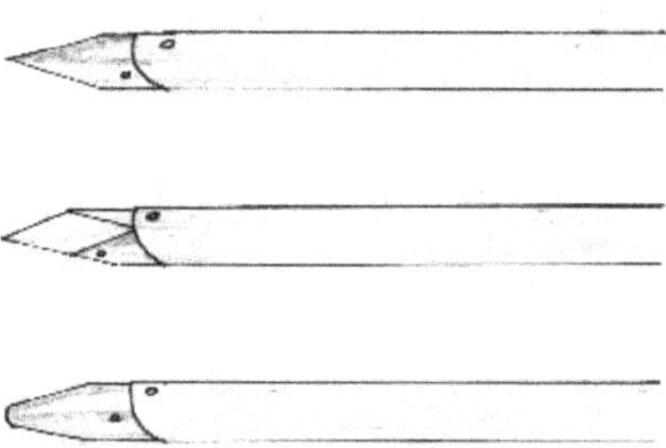

Because this type of trocar does not bleed from the insertion port. 2, 3, 4, etc. when inserting trocars into the abdominal cavity, we tried to insert them from the avascular areas of the abdominal wall (using the laparoscopic transillumination method).

Advanced methods used to prevent blood loss in other stages of SLOs are detailed in the above chapters.

Chronic anemia with iron deficiency was found in 35.22% (31) patients in our observations. All these were found to be iron deficiency anemia.

Chronic anemia was observed in 19 patients (61.29%) of the main group. 9 of these patients (50%) had mild, 6 (31.57%) moderate, and 4 (21.05%) severe chronic anemia.

According to the results of our determination of blood loss during these SLOs (measured on the scales of blood cells), the average blood loss did not exceed 30-60 ml in 95% of cases. The remaining 5% of patients had only 50-90 ml. In 2 cases, more bleeding from the gallbladder bed was observed after *LC* (around 150 mL) and was stopped with ultrasound coagulation. There were no cases of conversion due to bleeding.

According to the analysis of the above cases, performing SLOs with the help of improved laparoscopic technologies in patients suffering from chronic anemia and requiring surgical treatment, in addition to being less invasive and perfect surgical methods for patients, reduces the risks associated with the operation and the postoperative period. created the ground for its decrease. In patients with simultaneous abdominal pathologies that need to be treated by surgery, the occurrence of diseases of the cardiovascular system from concomitant therapeutic diseases causes specific problems in the treatment of these patients by surgery. It is known that among diseases of the cardiovascular system, myocardial infarction, cerebral stroke, and thromboembolic complications are common in these patients due to deep hemodynamic disorders (even in the absence of surgical trauma). Among the surgical and postoperative complications, hypoventilation syndrome, thromboembolic complications, wound suppuration, stroke, myocardial infarction are often observed in these patients. HD, obesity and diabetes often occur together. Now, taking into account the above, it is not difficult to imagine how dangerous it can be for patients to carry out simultaneous operations on abdominal organs in this category of patients. That is, as a result of simultaneous operations using traditional methods, as a result of the several times increase in the size of the operational injury caused to the patient, the cases of the occurrence of complications that are very dangerous for the patient's life will increase.

The information presented above shows that a number of problems arise in the surgical treatment of patients with diseases of the cardiovascular system and simultaneous abdominal pathologies. Caring for these patients in the pre-operation, operation and post-operation periods is of special importance and requires great responsibility.

During the study, diseases of the cardiovascular system were observed in 25 patients (20.45%). Among them, 21 (23.86%) patients had CKD, 4 (4.54%) patients had CKD (1 patient had a history of myocardial infarction, and 2 patients had a cerebral stroke). In 10 (11.36%) cases, SLOs such as separation of contracts with *LC*, LGP in 2 (2.27%), LTSE in 4 (4.54%) and LM in 2 (2.27%) cases were conducted. SLOs in these patients were performed preoperatively according to the cardiologist's recommendations, after eliminating the coronary syndrome with the help of fast and long-acting nitropreparations, the functional state of the myocardium, ECG, EcoCG, and physical tests were checked and positive changes were detected. It is of great importance that the stage of mental preparation of these patients for the operation is perfect.

Taking into account the effect of acidosis on the patient's body caused by the resorption of SO_2 gas during laparoscopy, the intra-abdominal gas pressure during SLO should be 7-9 mm. above and we ensured that the rate of gas entering the abdominal cavity did not exceed 0.15 l/s. If the patient's hemodynamic parameters did not change within the next 15 minutes, the operation was continued. During the entire operation, in order to prevent hypercapnia, an attempt was made to keep the SO_2 gas inlet rate at the above rate. It is ensured that the patient's head is raised up to 30-450.

The effect of induction anesthesia and pneumoperitoneum on reducing ABP was taken into account when conducting SLO in patients with HC. Intra-abdominal gas pressure should be increased by 10-12 mm. we ensured that it does not increase from At the same time, it has been proven that if the intra-abdominal gas pressure is too low, ABP may increase. It was clear from our observations that 10-12 mm of intra-abdominal gas pressure. above amount is the most optimal for these patients, and it will not be dangerous to change the patient's body position during the operation. A history of IM was not a contraindication for SLO.

Abdominal surgery in patients with adjacent somatic pathology, such as III-IV degree obesity, using traditional methods, causes a number of technical problems. III-IV degree obesity and pathologies such as IHD, HD occur together in almost all cases. In addition to thromboembolic and hypoventilation complications associated with the operation, such patients have a very high risk of developing complications such as myocardial infarction, brain stroke, wound suppuration, ligature fistulas, and postoperative hernias. In addition, due to the thickness of the abdominal wall, more blood is lost during the operation, in addition to technical difficulties, and as a result, the negative effects of the surgical wound increase. In the early days when endovisual technologies entered abdominal surgery, obesity of the III-IV degree was considered as a contraindication for surgery. But over time, the range of possibilities of these technologies has expanded, and nowadays operations are carried out with the help of laparoscopic technologies as much as possible in patients with obesity of the III-IV degree.

In our observations, it was found that 15 (17.04%) patients had III-IV degrees of obesity. Carrying out SLOs in such patients also has its own difficulties. These are: the thickness of the subcutaneous tissue and the front wall of the abdomen, the presence of deep functional and morphological changes in the cardiovascular and respiratory systems. Since hypoventilation syndrome was observed in the preoperative period (six patients had sleep apnea), the patients were given tranquilizers, sleeping pills, and narcotic analgesics. In order to prevent the mass in the stomach from falling into the respiratory tract, the patients were fed with small portions alternating with fasting for 12-16 hours, N2 blockers were given in the days before the operation.

In such patients, it is very difficult to puncture the anterior wall of the abdomen and create a pneumoperitoneum, to separate the bile duct, artery of the gallbladder, due to the large amount of fatty tissue in the hepatoduodenal ligament and the neck of the gallbladder. screams. For *LC*, inserting the first trocar above the umbilicus (because the abdomen is very large), and the second trocar of 10 mm in the epigastric area, from the edge of the round ligament of the liver, makes manipulations in the abdomen a little easier. After all trocars were inserted into the abdominal cavity, the position of the patient on the operating table was changed. The head side was raised up to 30-400, as a result, the intestines and large intestine were moved to the lower parts of the abdomen, the right side was raised to 300, and a better view of the area under the liver, where surgical manipulations were performed, was achieved. The left leg of the patient is raised to 35-400, which serves as a support for the patient on the operating table. Intra-abdominal gas pressure is 8-10 mm. We did not increase it, because it was observed that its increase over these indicators causes tachycardia and hypercapnia. In the initial period after the operation, the transfer of the patient's position to the Fowler's position had a good effect on the activity of the organs of the respiratory and cardiovascular system. Adhesion separation with *LC* in 6 (6.81%) patients, LTSE with *LC* in 4 (4.54%), LGP in 2 (2.27%) cases, LA in 1 (1.13%) case and 2 In 2 (2.27%) cases, *LESS* operations were performed. In order to facilitate and improve the transfer of *LC*, LA, LTSE from SLO stages in these patients (taking into account the thickness of the abdominal wall due to the subcutaneous fat layer), 2 P-shaped sutures (passing through all layers of the anterior abdominal wall) were used. With their help, the front wall of the abdomen was thinned to the maximum extent (up to 5-10 times). With the help of these threads, it was possible to move and sink the abdominal wall in the desired direction - up, down, right and left.

3.4. Analysis of results of simultaneous laparoscopic operations

In this group, we studied the results of all SLOs performed in simultaneous pathologies of the abdominal organs based on our observations during and after the operation: 1. General clinical observations (nausea, vomiting, intestinal paresis, pain the duration of the pain syndrome, etc. were studied). 2. Laboratory diagnostic procedures (blood smear analysis, determination of biochemical indicators, etc.). 3. Instrumental examinations (such as control USE, X-ray and endoscopic examinations). 4. Activation of patients - the beginning of vi.

Nausea and vomiting were observed in 26 (29.54%) patients on the first postoperative day. Intestinal paresis was observed in 15 (17.04%) patients and disappeared on the second postoperative day, in 7 (7.95%) cases after stimulation of bowel activity (proserin t/o and cleansing enema) disappeared.

All patients underwent blood tests for control in the postoperative period. Before removing the drainage tubes, the patients underwent USE. Examination with USE was also performed in patients with increased body temperature and severe pain syndrome after surgery. After the operation, the pain syndrome remained only on the first and second days, and it was enough to use non-narcotic analgesics to eliminate it. The description of postoperative indicators is shown in table 4.6.

4.6 Schedule

Description of postoperative indicators

Complications	Number
Need for analgesia	For 1-2 days
Nausea and vomiting	For 1-2days
Loss of intestinal parases	For 1-2days
The beginning of patient activation	1st -2nd day
Duration of the postoperative period,day	4,21±0,16
Teriostiem physema	2 (2,27%)
"Phrenicus syndrome"	2 (2,27%)
Separation of seroma	2 (2,27%)
Suppuration	1 (1,13%)

An exacerbation of chronic bronchitis	1 (1,13%)

Epigastric wound suppuration was observed in 1 (1.13%) case, seroma separation from the same wound in 2 (2.27%) cases, and subcutaneous emphysema in 2 (2.27%) patients. Subcutaneous emphysema resolved spontaneously within a week after surgery without any complications. A complication called "phrenicus syndrome", that is, a painful complication, was observed in 2 (2.27%) patients. The reason for this can be explained as the effect of pneumoperitoneum on the diaphragmatic nerve. These patients were bothered by pains under both ribs, which disappeared within a week. Chronic bronchitis was observed in 1 (1.13%) patient. Neither conversion nor death was observed among patients of this group.

In the postoperative period, independent movement and full activation were observed in 24 hours in 24 patients (Figure 4.11).

4.11 Figure

The graph of movement activity recovery of the main group of patients

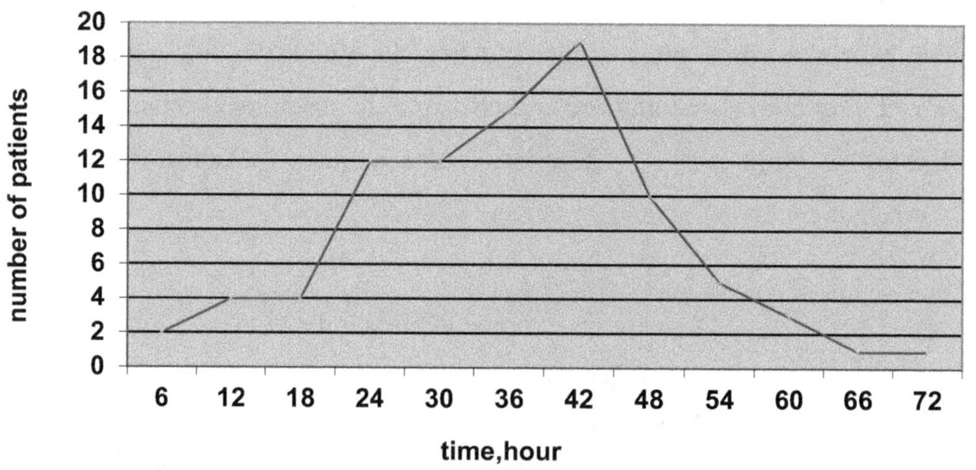

The average number of days of the patient's stay in the hospital was 6.03±0.22 days, and the postoperative period was 4.21±0.16 days.

Thus, in our study, the analysis of the results and complications recorded after SLOs in patients with a high risk of surgery (with concomitant therapeutic diseases) in our observations showed that abdominal organs in co-occurring pathologies, especially in patients with a high risk of surgery, that is, in patients with concomitant somatic diseases, as a result of the use of the improved options of SLOs proposed by us using laparoscopic technologies, the maximum reduction of postoperative complications was achieved.

Using the improved options of SLOs proposed by us, these operations are not only compared to traditional operations, but also from other types of SLOs. it is also distinguished by its economic, medical and social advantages.

Thus, patients with concomitant somatic diseases such as diseases of the cardiovascular system, anemia, III-IV degrees of obesity, which were contraindications for simultaneous surgery, before surgery on the organs of the abdominal cavity performed SLOs in patients with simultaneous surgical pathology found during the intraoperative period, the use of improved original methods laid the groundwork for the successful passage of operations and the expansion of the range of indications for them. It led to the achievement of high economic efficiency due to the reduction of temporary incapacity for work of patients and the reduction of expenses for treatment.

3.5. Comparative analysis of results of simultaneous laparoscopic operations

In the course of our study, a number of indicators were comparatively studied in both groups of patients in the pre-operation, operation and post-operation period. In the patients of the control group, there were no concomitant therapeutic diseases (except for chronic anemia) that aggravated the results of the operation, except for CSC and abdominal diseases. That is, the day before the operation, a light meal, cleaning injections in the evening and the morning of the operation, and, if necessary, sedatives were administered. Of course, general analyzes of blood, urine, feces, blood biochemical analysis, determination of blood group and rhesus factor, blood test for WR, USE, X-ray examinations, EGDFS, therapist and anesthesiologist consultations were also conducted.

The main group of patients, unlike the above (except CSC and CDAO, because they have concomitant therapeutic diseases that increase the risk of surgery), before the operation, the patients received medical treatments recommended by the necessary specialists (cardiologist, therapist, hematologist).

According to the classification proposed by D. Lohlein and Pichlmayr, in the control group, 22 small SLOs and 18 medium SLOs were included in simultaneous operations, while in the main group, all SLOs performed (48) were concomitant therapeutic diseases that increase the risk of surgery. was included in the series of heavy simultaneous operations.

During the operation, it is necessary to make specific improvements in the conditions of the operation table, in the formation of pneumoperitoneum and in maintaining it in the required state, in the selection of the operation method, among the main group of patients, and especially in patients with III-IV degree of obesity. came to mind (given in the above chapter).

When comparing the time spent on the operation, the following situation occurred (table 4.7).

A comparative view of the average duration of SLOs

Main stage	Simultaneous stage	Average duration of operation (minutes)	
		Control group	Main group
LC	separation of contracts	75,42±0,98	79,42±1,35*
LC	LESS	52,18±1,19	54,40±1,40
LC	LTSE	69,13±1,51	71,10±1,12
LC	LA	84,18±1,72	97,21±2,05*
LC	LH	81,66±1,67	93,73±2,15*
LC	Myomectomy	73,50±0,50	76,33±0,33*
LC	LTSE, LESS	64,40±1,07	79,40±1,76*
LC	LTSE, separation of contracts	92,41±1,35	106,40±1,52*

*Significance level R<0.05.

It can be seen from the table that when comparing the time spent on SLO, LC and LTSE, on average 92.41±1.35 minutes were spent in the control group to separate the contracts, while in the main group it was 106.40 ±1.52 minutes spent, 14 minutes more. For LC and LA, 84.18±1.72 minutes were spent in the control group, 97.21±2.05 minutes in the main group. No significant difference was observed in the time spent on conducting other types of SLOs.

A comparative description of the indicators after the conducted SLO is given in table 4.8.

Comparative description of postoperative indicators

Name	Control group		Main group	
	indicators	%	indicators	%
Analgesia	for 1-2 days	-	for 1-2 days	-
Nausea and vomiting	on the 1st day	-	for 1-2 days	-
Loss of intestinal paresis	for 1-2 days	-	for 1-2 days	-
Patient activation	on the 1st	-	on the 1st and 2nd	-

	day		days	
Duration of the postoperative period, day	3,88±0,14	-	4,21±0,16	-
Subcutaneous emphysema	2	2,50	2	2,27
Phrenicus syndrome	2	2,50	2	2,27
Separation of seroma	1	1,25	2	2,27
Suppuration	1	1,25	1	1,13
Provocation of chronic bronchitis	-	-	1	1,13

When analyzing postoperative complications such as wound suppuration, seroma separation, subcutaneous emphysema, "phrenicus syndrome", despite the fact that patients of the main group had concomitant therapeutic diseases that increase the risk of surgery, the results of their treatment were maximally close to those of the control group.

In the control group, 21 (26.25%) patients had nausea and vomiting on the first postoperative day. Intestinal paresis was observed in 11 (13.75%) patients and resolved spontaneously by the second postoperative day, while in 5 (6.25%) patients it disappeared after bowel stimulation. .

Among the main group of patients, nausea and vomiting were observed in 26 (29.54%) patients on the first postoperative day, intestinal paresis was observed in 15 (17.04%) patients on the second postoperative day, and 7 (7, 95%) disappeared after stimulation of bowel activity (proserin t/o and cleansing enema).
Conversion and death were not observed in both groups.

The average number of days in the hospital of the patients of the control group was 5.85±0.22 days, and the postoperative period was 3.88±0.14 days.

This indicator was as follows in the main group: the average number of days in the hospital was 6.03±0.22 days, and the postoperative period was 4.21±0.16 days.

In the control group, 36 hours after the operation, the general condition of all patients was satisfactory. 6 (7.50%) patients were able to move independently 6 hours after the operation and were allowed to go home the next day. Full activation of independent movement was observed in 58 patients within 24 hours, while independent movement and full activation was observed in 56 patients in the main group within 24 hours (Figure 4.12).

4.12 Figure

The graph of movement activity recovery of control and main group patients

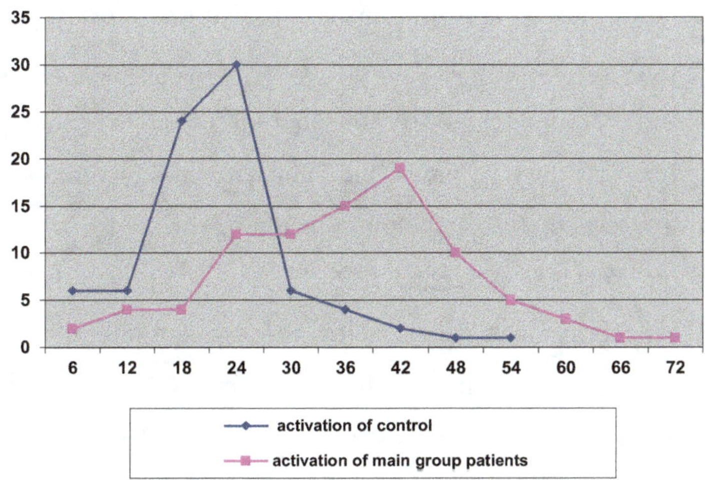

Therefore, as a result of using the improved methods of SLOs proposed by us, it was achieved that the results of SLOs performed in patients with a high risk of surgery are no worse than the results of SLOs performed in patients of the control group.

CONCLUSION

Chronic cholecystitis (CC) is one of the most common diseases in the world today. If this disease occurs in 10-15% of the world's population and this rate doubles on average every 10 years, it is predicted that it will become the main problem in the field of surgical gastroenterology by the second half of the 21st century. . In addition to the high incidence of this disease among the elderly and elderly population, this category of patients has a high risk of surgery, and there are many cases of deterioration of the results of the operation due to age and related therapeutic pathologies. Surgery remains the main method of treating chronic stone cholecystitis, especially its complicated types. However, complications after traditional surgical procedures (5-26%) and climate index remain high (0.3-25.5%), especially in patients with concomitant therapeutic diseases that increase the risk of surgery. In patients older than 60 years, it is predicted that the climate index will increase by 2-3 times every next 10 years. As a result of the experience gained in recent years, the improvement of surgical techniques and equipment, not only the psychology of surgeons, but also the attitude of patients to the operation methods is changing, that is, the desire to get rid of all their diseases at the same time is increasing. Regarding the need to improve the types of surgical treatment of chronic stone cholecystitis in patients with a risk of surgery, it is known from the above data that two or more diseases that require surgical treatment at the same time in the patients encountered, especially in almost the majority of cases, not only simultaneous operations, but also in the case of patients with common concomitant therapeutic diseases, which hinder the conduct of simple operations, sharply increase the risk of surgery, using new, modern technologies, which cause less damage to the patient's body , conducting scientific research in modern abdominal surgery in order to apply operative treatment methods that are low-cost, have a high cosmetic result, are convenient, quick and easier for patients to undergo mentally, to improve existing ones, to create new ones and to put them into practice It is one of the most well-known needs, which is not only theoretical, but also of great practical importance.

Based on the above, the aim of the study is to improve the methods of simultaneous laparoscopic surgery in patients with a high risk of surgery.

To realize our goal, we set ourselves the following tasks:

1. Improving methods of simultaneous laparoscopic surgery in patients with a high risk of surgery, when simultaneous pathologies of abdominal organs are observed together with chronic stone cholecystitis.

2. To study the results of operations improved by laparoscopic technologies in patients with a high risk of surgery and co-occurring diseases of abdominal organs.

3. Comparative study of the results of simultaneous laparoscopic operations in patients with a high risk of surgery.

Our research work is based on the results of treatment of 88 patients who underwent SLO in patients with high risk of surgery and chronic cholecystitis. From 2019 to 2023, these patients received operative treatment in the Department of Endosurgery (Thoracic Surgery) of the Khorezm Region Multidisciplinary Medical Center.

The conducted SLOs were divided according to severity levels according to the classification proposed by D. Lo'lein and Pichlmayr (1978):

1. Small simultaneous operations, operations that do not greatly increase the operational injury and operational risk;

2. Medium-level operations, operations that increase the surgical injury, but do not significantly increase the risk of the operation;

3. Operations with a high level of operational risk, operations in cases of surgical injury and conditions that sharply increase the risk of operation, concomitant diseases are observed

Our scientific research work was based on the results of treatment of 88 patients with CSC and CDAO who underwent SLO. These patients were treated in the endosurgery departments of the Khorezm Regional Multidisciplinary Medical Center from 2018 to 2023.

91.07% of the studied patients were women. The number of men was 8 and made up 8.92%. More than 85% of patients were aged between 20 and 60 years, and 11 (13.09%) were older than 60 years.

When the anamnesis information about CSC infection was collected from the patients, we obtained the following results:

Anamnesis up to 1 year was found in 8 (13.33%) patients, anamnesis up to 3 years in 16 (30.77%) patients, and anamnesis up to 5 years and more in 28 (46.67%) patients.

The most frequently performed SLO was LC and adhesion separation surgery and was performed in 20 (22.72%) cases. LESS with LC was performed in 13 (14.77%) patients, LTSE in 12 (13.63%) patients, LA in 9 (10.22%) patients, LH in 11 (12.5%) patients, and LM in 5 (5.68%) patients.

As a result of the introduction of endovisual technology into practice, it became possible to perform three, four and even five pathologies at the same time in abdominal organs, which are almost impossible to perform with traditional methods. During our study, we performed such operations in 29 (32.95%) patients.

The results of the treatment of the patients were divided into 2 groups.

40 patients who underwent SLO were included in the control group. In this group of patients, there were no concomitant therapeutic diseases that significantly increase the risk of surgery in addition to CSC and affect its results. 48 patients who underwent SLO were included in the main group. In addition to CSC, patients of this group have concomitant therapeutic diseases that increase the risk of surgery and affect its results (moderate and severe levels of chronic anemia, III-IV levels of obesity, IHD, HD) and abdominal cavity a cases such as previous surgery have been observed.

The conducted SLOs were divided according to the severity levels according to the classification proposed by D. Lohlein and Pichlmayr (1978):

1. Small simultaneous operations, operations that do not greatly increase the injury and risk of operation;

2. Medium-level operations, operations that increase the injury of the operation, but do not significantly increase the risk of the operation;

3. Operations with a high level of operational risk, operations in cases where the risk of surgical injury and operation is sharply increased, concomitant diseases are observed.

Out of 40 SLOs performed in control group patients, 18 small and 22 medium simultaneous operations were included.

48 SLOs performed in the main group of patients were included in simultaneous operations with a high operational risk.

Preoperative preparation of all patients consisted of a light meal the day before surgery, evening and morning cleansing enemas, and traditional premedication 30 minutes before surgery.

The main group of patients followed the advice of the necessary specialists (hematologist, therapist, cardiologist, anesthesiologist) in the pre-operative period and received all the treatments recommended by them.

During our study, we used several improved versions of SLOs performed in the control and main groups: in the control group, we used more traditional methods, and in the main group, we used a movable L-shaped electrode to separate adhesions with LC. When performing LA with LC, in all cases, after LC was performed in the standard way, we used an improved variant of LA (and in the control group, we used variants 1-4). We used 2 methods of LH in both groups of patients.

LESS was carried out in 5 options together with elimination of the main pathology.

It is worth noting that almost 70% of all patients under our observation during the study were women of reproductive age, and 37 of them asked us to perform IJS laparoscopically after the necessary explanations. Because these women had contraindications to other types of contraception.

During our scientific research, we improved and put into practice 7 new laparoscopic surgery methods.

If we take into account the fact that 90% of the population living in the Lower Arolbay region suffer from chronic anemia, there is no doubt how dangerous it is for this category of patients to perform simultaneous operations with traditional methods. In patients with moderate and severe levels of chronic anemia, not only the specifics of the preparatory stage in the preoperative period (hematologist's consultation, hemotransfusion, etc.), is related to the direct operation, but also to anesthesia, the passage of the postoperative period (healing of the wound , volume of treatment procedures, hemotransfusion, etc.) a number of problems may arise.

All patients with chronic anemia followed the hematologist's recommendations and received blood, blood substitutes, hemopoiesis-improving, vitamin, and iron preparations before surgery.

In the control group, 12 (38.7%) of the total patients had chronic iron deficiency anemia, of which 6 (50.0%) had mild, 4 (33.34%) moderate, and 2 (16.66%) severe anemia. . Although 34 patients had moderate and severe levels of chronic anemia, SLOs were fulfilled.

Chronic anemia with iron deficiency was observed in 19 patients (61.29%) in the main group. 9 of these patients (50%) had mild, 6 (33.34%) moderate, and 4 (16.67%) severe chronic anemia. Although 10 patients had moderate and severe levels of chronic anemia, SLOs were fulfilled.

During the study, diseases of the cardiovascular system were observed in 25 (20.45%) of the main group of patients. Among them: 18 (13.63%) patients had CKD, 4 (6.81%) patients had CKD (1 patient had a history of myocardial infarction, and 2 patients had a cerebral stroke).

These patients were examined in the pre-operative period after coronary syndrome was eliminated with the help of fast and long-acting nitropreparations according to the recommendations of the cardiologist, the functional condition of the myocardium, ECG, EcoCG, and physical tests were examined and positive changes were detected. It is of great importance that the stage of mentally preparing these patients for the operation is perfect.

In our observations, 14 (15.90%) patients in the main group had III-IV degrees of obesity. Carrying out SLOs in such patients also has its own difficulties. These are: the thickness of the subcutaneous tissue and the front wall of the abdomen, the presence of deep functional and morphological changes in the cardiovascular and respiratory systems.

During our observations, it was found that 8 (16.67%) patients in the main group had previous surgery in their anamnesis. Of these, 2 (4.16%) had acute appendicitis (complicated with diffuse peritonitis), 2 (4.16%) had large anterior abdominal wall hernias, 2 (4.16%) had ovarian cysts, 1 had peptic ulcer disease, and 1 had uterine fibroids. it became known that they conducted an operation on These data and the scars on the anterior abdominal wall were taken into account at the site of abdominal puncture in SLOs.

The following indicators were analyzed in order to assess the tissue damage and the general condition of patients in SLOs:

1. Dimensions of the path to the operated organ (the number of holes in the front wall of the abdomen);

2. Post-operative period (general condition of patients, complaints, results of objective examination, paresis of intestines, length of stay of drainage tubes, etc.);

4. Results of laboratory and instrumental examinations in the postoperative period (USE, X-ray examination, endoscopic examinations, general and biochemical indicators of blood, etc.);

5. The number of anesthesia in the postoperative period;

6. Beginning of patient activation;

7. Number of days;

8. Medicine - consumption of medicine, sewing and bandage materials;

9. The ability of patients to carry out the operation mentally;

10. Cosmetic efficiency.

In order to comprehensively evaluate the general condition of patients, to make a comparative diagnosis of various pathologies, the following examinations were carried out:

1. Clinical examinations: collecting complaints and anamnesis, general examination, palpation of the chest and abdomen, percussion, pulse and control of ABP.

2. Laboratory examination of blood and urine: general analyzes of blood and urine, blood coagulation and coagulogram, bilirubin, determination of transferases, urea, blood sugar, diastase, creatinine, nitrogen metabolism, blood biochemical parameters such as total protein.

3. ECG.

4. Ultrasound examination of the liver and bile ducts, pancreas, spleen, kidneys, lower part of the abdominal cavity, small pelvic organs (on the SSD-630 ultrasound scanner of the Japanese firm "Aloka").

5. EGDFS (with an endoscope CF-10 model of the Japanese company "Olympus").

6. General radiography of the chest and abdomen.

7. X-ray examination of the gastrointestinal tract.

8. Gynecologist examination and advice.

9. Examination and consultation of therapist, anesthesiologist.

All laparoscopic operations were performed under general intubation anesthesia using endosurgical equipment such as "Tantorro" (Germany) and ultrasonic scalpel "Hormonic". The intensity of the light flow was controlled by manual and automatic lighting system devices. We created the pneumoperitoneum with the help of an insufflator with an electronic control system using SO_2 and nitrogen (II) oxide gases. In the second group, in patients with IHD, HD, III-IV degrees of obesity from additional somatic diseases, pneumoperitoneum was created very carefully, in the case of pneumoperitoneum as small as possible (the pressure in the abdominal cavity was reduced by 8-10 mm of wire .without exceeding) SLOs met. An electronic coagulator working in high-frequency "cutting" and "coagulation" mode was used to separate tissues or stop blood. In order to achieve reliable hemostasis during LC in patients with severe chronic anemia, ultrasonic coagulation using the URSK - 7N - 22 device was used.

The complications observed during the study were divided into 3 groups (according to T.B. Duboshina, 1980):

1. Complications related to the performed operations:

a) special (specific)

b) non-specific

2. Complications related to the main pathology.

3. Complications related to concomitant pathology.

The analysis of the received data and statistical processing of numerical indicators was carried out on the "Pentium-IV" computer based on the "Excel" and Access (Microsoft, USA) system programs.

The level of accuracy of the main indicators for groups was determined using the Fisher-Student test. We considered indicators with a difference in the level of compatibility of less than 0.5% ($p<0.05$) to be accurate.

In all cases, the main phase of SLOs, which were also performed in the main group, was organized by LC. In 20 (23.86%) cases, the main pathology was observed together with abdominal adhesion disease. Because this condition is often located around the gallbladder, scrotal tumor, ovaries, and other organs, patients with CSC , on inquiry, in addition to right subcostal pain, gastrointestinal discomfort, that is, nausea, vomiting, flatulence, flatulence and other similar complaints were observed. It was found that these complaints were formed due to the adhesion of the transverse colon, duodenum, stomach and other organs to the adhesion process around the gallbladder.

In 6 (6.81%) patients, the bulbous part of the duodenum and the pyloric canal, the large intestine were attached to the Hartmann's pouch of the gall bladder, and in 3 patients, the rest of the stomach and the duodenum, the hepatoduodenal ligament were completely attached to this area. it was found that the big car that he had closed was stuck. In order to prevent iatrogenic damage to the pyloric canal and duodenum, it was necessary to separate adhesions not only from the gallbladder wall, but also from its serous layer.

Carrying out SLOs in patients who have previously undergone surgery on the organs of the abdominal cavity has gained special importance and caused specific difficulties. This is especially observed when there is a postoperative scar on the white line of the abdomen near the navel. It was found that 15 (17.04%) patients had previous surgery in their anamnesis. Of these, 6 (6.81%) had acute appendicitis (complicated with diffuse peritonitis), 3 (3.41%) had large anterior abdominal wall hernias, 4 (45.45%) had ovarian cysts, and 1 had gastric ulcer disease. , 1 was found to have undergone an operation for uterine myoma. In such patients, it is very important to enter the Veresh needle and the first trocar into the abdominal cavity. Because there is a high risk of uncontrolled insufflation of gas into the abdominal cavity and injury to the hollow organs. In our opinion, it would be correct to determine the most convenient point for puncture and the first trocar in these patients from the left flank area, because adhesion process was observed the least after previous open operations in this area. The remaining points are made from the most convenient areas under the control of a laparoscope.

We selected the first point for creating a pneumoperitoneum and serving as a port for the laparoscope individually for each patient. It was taken into account the degree of development of the subcutaneous tissue, the previous operation, and the presence of signs of intestinal obstruction due to adhesions. Since 18 (35,23) patients did not have umbilical hernia or postoperative scars in this area, we chose point 1a below the navel as the first point. In patients with umbilical hernia or postoperative scars below the umbilicus along the white line of the abdomen (5.7 and 2.8%), we used point 1b above the umbilicus to enter with a trocar.

This point was also used in patients with IV degree obesity. After inserting a laparoscope into the abdominal cavity from the first point, the abdominal cavity was examined in detail. Further tactics depended on the results of the inspection. If adhesions were found in the subhepatic and hepatoduodenal areas, the second manipulator was inserted into the abdominal cavity from the right flank (8 cases). Entered from the area under a (in 3 cases). As a result of the location of the attachment process on the upper floor of the abdominal cavity, we had to use the second manipulator in 3 cases to the left of the navel, from the lateral edge of the rectus muscle, and in 7 cases to the same point on the right side. Usually, manipulators inserted from two 5-mm trocars are sufficient to separate adhesions, but in 5 cases it was necessary to insert 3 x 5-mm trocars. After the formation of pneumoperitoneum, adhesions formed between large intestine, intestines and anterior abdominal wall become visible and easy to separate. In 11 of 21 such patients, it was found that the anterior abdominal wall, large intestine, transverse colon and liver were involved in the adhesion process. In cases of obesity of the IV degree and a lot of fatty tissue in the round neck of the liver (6.38%), we introduced the main manipulator from point 2b. A 10-mm trocar is inserted through the lateral edge of the round ligament of the liver, making it easier to work in the subhepatic area. Therefore, it is advisable to plan all the procedures to be performed in advance and use the holes made in the front wall of the abdomen. Separation of contracts using the above-mentioned methods has its own disadvantages. For example, it takes a lot of time to separate adhesions, the reliability of hemostasis is not high. Therefore, we used these methods only at the beginning of our research. Later, we created a "mobile" L-shaped electrode that facilitates the cutting of adhesions in the abdominal cavity and used it in 21 patients. In cases of advanced adhesions, the time of separation of adhesions is reduced by several times as a result of the use of a "mobile" L-shaped electrode, reliable hemostasis is achieved and separation of adhesions becomes easier, because in this case adhesions are "collected" and brought to a state of compression and cut in place, tearing of the serous layer of the intestine (deserosis), complications such as bleeding are not observed

Usually, we start LC as far from the choledox as possible, in the neck of the gallbladder. After identification of the bile duct of the gallbladder, it is clipped. In cases where the normal clip does not fit the gall bladder artery (in its band type) (in 7 patients), it is separated from the maximally close places to the gall bladder with the help of an L-shaped electrode with a coagulator. After the gall bladder is separated, if there are signs of bleeding from its place, coagulation is performed with the help of clamp or shovel electrodes.

During our study, skin incisions, intra-abdominal insertion of trocars, tissue dissection, gallbladder artery and bile duct clipping, gallbladder dissection and replacement were performed. we developed a new method. This method consists in cutting the skin with an ultrasound knife with a low-frequency resonant vibration frequency of 23.9-26.9 kHz, a power of 0.2-0.4 W/cm2 and a current of 6-8 mA (invention received a preliminary patent from the State Patent Office, IDP 04858). An ultrasound scalpel with a length of 20-50 cm and a diameter of 5-10 mm, equipped with a special waveguide, is inserted into the abdominal cavity through the epigastric port, and the gallbladder is treated with it. Point ultrasound coagulation is continued from top to bottom until a thin but strong film is formed. CSC and chronic appendicitis were found together in 9 (10.22%) cases. When the complaints and anamnesis of patients with this CSC were analyzed in depth and purposefully, it was noted that in addition to the typical anamnesis and complaints of this disease, they also have pains in the right flank area that appear from time to time, often of a radiating nature. . Chronic appendicitis is suspected in patients with such complaints. Because these patients were informed about the possibilities of laparoscopic technologies, they also agreed to LA operation together with LC. In these patients, during diagnostic laparoscopy, there are adhesions in the area of the vermiform tumor and signs of chronic inflammation of the tumor (deformation, uneven thickening of the walls of the vermiform tumor, focal hypertrophy, signs of atrophy, etc.) is planned to be held.

The technique of performing simultaneous LC and LA was as follows: 1 and 2 x 10 mm trocars and 3 x 5 mm trocars were inserted from the standard points while inserting the trocars into the abdominal cavity for LC surgery, taking into account the LA stage. if inserted, instead of the 4th 5 mm trocar, a 10 mm trocar was inserted from the right flank area through the Mac Burney point. Other stages of LC were performed in the usual conventional manner. Then the laparoscope was moved to the port in the epigastric area. Then, an additional 5 mm trocar was inserted from the left side, and the patient's position was changed to that of the LTSE operation, and the right side was raised to 15-200. We used several traditional variants of LA in the initial stages of our study and in control group patients. These methods have been used more and more to perform single LAs, allowing to select the most convenient options as a stage of SLO and to be performed not only together with LC, but also with other laparoscopic operations (LTSE, LH, separation of adhesions). . We used LC and LA together in several options, improving the methods used in control group patients and eliminating their shortcomings.

Abdominal white line and umbilical hernias were observed in 15 (17.04%) patients together with CSC, and the size of the hernia gate was greater than 4 cm. LH was performed together with LC in these patients. The hernia gate was closed with a special polypropylene mesh and eliminated. The execution technique is as follows: The skin and subcutaneous tissue over the hernia is cut longitudinally or transversely by 1.5-2 cm. When the hernia sac was found, it was opened and the organ inside was determined to be viable, then it was inserted into the abdominal cavity. Then a 10 mm trocar was inserted into the abdominal cavity from this place and sealed with 2-4 stitches. The LC phase of the SLO was performed in the usual way. Then, a pre-prepared polypropylene mesh was inserted into the abdominal cavity from the trocar in the epigastric region to close the hernial gate (when the hernial gate is larger than 4 cm). The size of the mesh should be 2-4 cm wide and 2 cm longer than the size of the hernial gate (after straightening). On the edges of the net there are 8 to 12 lavsan threads, 15-20 cm long, which are easily pulled out with a hook needle. The distance between the threads should not be greater than 15-20 mm. So that the threads do not get tangled, the edge of the net was tied with the help of thin kapron threads. After being inserted into the abdominal cavity, the mesh was straightened and brought to the area of the hernial gate with a clamp. Then, the lavsan threads on the edge of the mesh were pulled under the skin with the help of a hooked needle. In this case, the needle should enter the abdominal cavity 2 cm away from the edge of the hernial gate. After pulling out all the threads, they were tied under the skin (over the aponeurosis). With this method, the polypropylene mesh was attached to the hernial gate without too much tension and the hernial gate was eliminated. All the manipulations listed above were performed under strict laparoscope control.

Since the majority of CSC patients are women, it was necessary to pay special attention to their gynecological conditions during preoperative examinations. Cystectomy surgery was performed laparoscopically in all patients (12 patients) who were diagnosed with an ovarian cyst with LC. Patients were examined by a gynecologist in the pre-operative period and an indication for cystectomy was determined. In these patients, we performed the LC stage of SLO in the order indicated above. When choosing the points for trocars, the side of the cyst, the body structure of the patients, and previous surgery were taken into account. After performing the LC stage of SLO, the position of the patient on the operating table was changed, i.e., the head side was raised 20 - 250 degrees down, the leg side was raised 25 - 300 degrees. Depending on the size, character, and location of the cyst (on the leg, adherent, intraligamentary, etc.), the LTSE stage of SLO was performed as follows.

As a result of our use of LTSEs of the above variants in the elimination of ovarian cysts in the early stages of our study and in patients of the control group, it became clear that these variants are not without their own shortcomings. That is, despite the fact that in the first option presented in chapter 3, less time is spent on removing the cyst, and it is a less traumatic and organ-preserving operation method, the probability of cyst re-formation (recurrence) is higher. taking into account that it takes more time and is technically more complicated, and the fourth option was difficult to perform in patients with III-IV obesity, we used the improved option of LTSE. After the LC stage of SLO, regardless of the size of the ovarian cyst, it was punctured under the control of a laparoscope and the liquid inside was aspired. Then the laparoscope was moved from the paraumbilical port to the epigastric port.

In 13 patients (17.04%) who were infected with CSC and had indications for LSS, LESS operation with LC was performed. LESS was guided by women's wishes and the presence of contraindications to other types of contraception.

Taking into account that the LESS stage of the simultaneous operation can be easily performed from the trocar insertion points required for the LC stage, the first trocar was inserted as usual from the paraumbilical area. In women with normosthenic and asthenic body structure (9), 2nd, 3rd, 4th trocars were inserted into the abdominal cavity, taking into account the planned LC and LSS. That is, the 2nd trocar was inserted from the epigastric area, the 3rd trocar was inserted from the right subcostal area, and the 4th trocar was inserted from the right flank area. In patients with III-IV degree of obesity (6), one of the 5-mm trocars had to be inserted slightly lower than in the previous cases, and in 4 cases, the analog trocar had to be inserted from the left iliac region. . After completing the main stages of LC, we transferred the laparoscope from the parumbilical port to the epigastric port and changed the position of the patient on the operating table. That is, if we raised the lower part of the body by 30-400, we lowered the head. This situation led to the displacement of the intestines and large intestine to the upper parts of the abdominal cavity and improved visibility in the pelvic cavity. Once the fallopian tubes were identified, their occlusion was performed in the following manner. In contrast to the 4 methods presented in the above chapter, this method is much easier, faster and more reliable in terms of execution technique, in which the position of the patient on the operating table is changed after the LC stage of SLO is performed. Then a segment of the fallopian tube was cut from the place closest to the uterus by coagulation using a bipolar coagulator (in 11 cases).

Simultaneous LC and myomectomy was performed in 5 (5.68%) patients. In these patients, it was found that the myomatous nodes were located in the subserosal area and their size was not larger than 9 weeks, and they were an indication for laparoscopic myomectomy. After LC, which is the main stage of SLO, we changed the position of the patient on the operating table to that of LTSE. An additional 10-mm trocar was inserted into the abdominal cavity from the left side. Then, using bipolar coagulation, we separated the myomatous node from the surrounding tissues.

One of the main factors preventing the desired surgical treatment, especially operations on the abdominal organs, is the patient's (apart from surgical pathologies) and today's common concomitant therapeutic diseases. Chronic anemia ranks first among these diseases. That is why this category of patients is still at a high risk of performing simultaneous operations at CDAO. Especially, such a situation is clearly reflected in the surgical removal of CSC patients and pathologies of the pelvic organs. In order to eliminate such simultaneous pathologies through existing traditional open methods, it is necessary to expand the upper middle laparotomy incision or to make a separate incision for cholecystectomy, to eliminate pelvic cavity pathology. As a result of this, it is natural to lose a lot of blood, in simple uncomplicated cholecystectomy or appendectomy operations, blood loss ranges from 100 ml to 500 ml, while in simultaneous operations, this figure is at least twice as much.

Advanced methods used to prevent blood loss in other stages of SLOs are detailed in the above chapters.

Chronic anemia with iron deficiency was found in 35.22% (31) patients in our observations. All these were found to be iron deficiency anemia.

Chronic anemia was observed in 19 patients (61.29%) of the main group. 9 of these patients (50%) had mild, 6 (31.57%) moderate, and 4 (21.05%) severe chronic anemia.

According to the results of our determination of blood loss during these SLOs (measured on the scales of blood cells), the average blood loss did not exceed 30-60 ml in 95% of cases. The remaining 5% of patients had only 50-90 ml. In 2 cases, more bleeding from the gallbladder bed was observed after LC (around 150 mL) and was stopped with ultrasound coagulation. There were no cases of conversion due to bleeding.

According to the analysis of the above cases, performing SLOs with the help of improved laparoscopic technologies in patients suffering from chronic anemia and requiring surgical treatment, in addition to being less invasive and perfect surgical methods for patients, reduces the risks associated with the operation and the postoperative period. created the ground for its decrease.

In patients with simultaneous abdominal pathologies that need to be treated by surgery, the occurrence of diseases of the cardiovascular system from concomitant therapeutic diseases causes specific problems in the treatment of these patients by surgery. It is known that among diseases of the cardiovascular system, myocardial infarction, cerebral stroke, and thromboembolic complications are common in these patients due to deep hemodynamic disorders (even in the absence of surgical trauma). Among the surgical and postoperative complications, hypoventilation syndrome, thromboembolic complications, wound suppuration, stroke, myocardial infarction are often observed in these patients. HD obesity and diabetes often occur together. Now, taking into account the above, it is not difficult to imagine how dangerous it can be for patients to carry out simultaneous operations on abdominal organs in this category of patients. That is, as a result of simultaneous operations using traditional methods, as a result of the several times increase in the size of the operational injury caused to the patient, the cases of the occurrence of complications that are very dangerous for the patient's life will increase.

The information presented above shows that a number of problems arise in the surgical treatment of patients with diseases of the cardiovascular system and simultaneous abdominal pathologies. Caring for these patients in the pre-operation, operation and post-operation periods is of special importance and requires great responsibility.

During the study, diseases of the cardiovascular system were observed in 25 patients (20.45%). Of these, 21 (23.86%) patients had CKD, 4 (4.54%) patients had CKD (1 patient had a history of myocardial infarction, and 2 patients had a cerebral stroke). In 10 (11.36%) cases, SLOs such as separation of contracts with LC, LH in 2 (2.27%), LTSE in 4 (4.54%) and LM in 2 (2.27%) cases were conducted. .

SLOs in these patients were performed preoperatively according to the cardiologist's recommendations, after eliminating the coronary syndrome with the help of fast and long-acting nitropreparations, the functional state of the myocardium, ECG, EcoCG, and physical tests were checked and positive changes were detected. It is of great importance that the stage of mental preparation of these patients for the operation is perfect.

Taking into account the effect of acidosis on the patient's body caused by the resorption of SO2 gas during laparoscopy, the intra-abdominal gas pressure during SLO should be 7-9 mm. above and we ensured that the rate of gas entering the abdominal cavity did not exceed 0.15 l/s. If the patient's hemodynamic parameters did not change within the next 15 minutes, the operation was continued. During the entire operation, in order to prevent hypercapnia, an attempt was made to keep the SO2 gas inlet rate at the above rate. It is ensured that the patient's head is raised up to 30-450.

The effect of induction anesthesia and pneumoperitoneum on reducing ABP was taken into account when conducting SLO in patients with HC. In order to prevent a sharp decrease in ABP during the operation, we ensured that the intra-abdominal gas pressure did not exceed 10-12 mm Hg. At the same time, it has been proven that if the intra-abdominal gas pressure is too low, ABP may increase. It was clear from our observations that 10-12 mm of intra-abdominal gas pressure. above amount is the most optimal for these patients, and it will not be dangerous to change the patient's body position during the operation. A history of IM was not a contraindication for SLO.

Abdominal surgery in patients with adjacent somatic pathology, such as III-IV obesity, using traditional methods, causes a number of technical problems. III-IV degree obesity and pathologies such as IHD, HD occur together in almost all cases. In addition to thromboembolic and hypoventilation complications associated with surgery, such patients have a very high risk of developing complications such as myocardial infarction, brain stroke, wound suppuration, ligature fistulae, and postoperative hernias. In addition, due to the thickness of the abdominal wall, more blood is lost during the operation, in addition to technical difficulties, and as a result, the negative effects of the surgical wound increase.

In the early days when endovisual technologies entered abdominal surgery, obesity of the III-IV degree was considered as a contraindication for surgery. But over time, the range of possibilities of these technologies has expanded, and nowadays operations are carried out with the help of laparoscopic technologies as much as possible in patients with obesity of the III-IV degree.

In our observations, it was found that 15 (17.04%) patients had III-IV degrees of obesity. Carrying out SLOs in such patients also has its own difficulties. These are: the thickness of the subcutaneous tissue and the front wall of the abdomen, the presence of deep functional and morphological changes in the cardiovascular and respiratory systems. Since hypoventilation syndrome was observed in the preoperative period (six patients had sleep apnea), the patients were given tranquilizers, sleeping pills, and narcotic analgesics. In order to prevent the mass in the stomach from falling into the respiratory tract, the patients were fed with small portions alternating with fasting for 12-16 hours, N2 blockers were given in the days before the operation.

In such patients, it is very difficult to puncture the anterior wall of the abdomen and create a pneumoperitoneum, divide the bile duct and artery of the gallbladder, due to the large amount of fatty tissue in the hepatoduodenal ligament and the neck of the gallbladder. screams. For LC, inserting the first trocar above the umbilicus (because the abdomen is very large), and the second trocar of 10 mm in the epigastric area, from the edge of the round ligament of the liver, makes manipulations in the abdomen a little easier. After all trocars were inserted into the abdominal cavity, the position of the patient on the operating table was changed. The head side was raised up to 30-400, as a result, the intestines and large intestine were moved to the lower parts of the abdomen, the right side was raised to 300, and a better view of the area under the liver, where surgical manipulations were performed, was achieved. The left leg of the patient is raised to 35-400, which serves as a support for the patient on the operating table. Intra-abdominal gas pressure is 8-10 mm. We did not increase it, because it was observed that its increase over these indicators causes tachycardia and hypercapnia. In the initial period after the operation, the transfer of the patient's position to Fowler's position had a good effect on the activity of the organs of the respiratory and cardiovascular systems.

In this group, we studied the results of all SLOs performed in simultaneous pathologies of the abdominal organs based on our observations during and after the operation: 1. General clinical observations (nausea, vomiting, intestinal paresis, pain the duration of the pain syndrome, etc. were studied). 2. Laboratory diagnostic procedures (blood smear analysis, determination of biochemical parameters, etc.). 3. Instrumental examinations (such as control USE, X-ray and endoscopic examinations). 4. Patient activation is the beginning of vi.

Nausea and vomiting were observed in 26 (29.54%) patients on the first postoperative day. Intestinal paresis was observed in 15 (17.04%) patients and disappeared on the second postoperative day, in 7 (7.95%) cases after stimulation of bowel activity (proserin t/o and cleansing enema) disappeared.

All patients underwent blood tests for control in the postoperative period. Before removing drainage tubes, patients underwent USE. Examination with USE was also performed in patients with increased body temperature and severe pain syndrome after surgery. After the operation, the pain syndrome remained only on the first and second days, and it was enough to use non-narcotic analgesics to eliminate it.

In the postoperative period, 24 patients had independent movement and full activation within 24 hours.

The average number of days of the patient's stay in the hospital was 6.03±0.22 days, and the postoperative period was 4.21±0.16 days.

Thus, in our study, the analysis of the results and complications recorded after SLOs in patients with a high risk of surgery (with concomitant therapeutic diseases) in our observations showed that abdominal organs in co-occurring pathologies, especially in patients with a high risk of surgery, that is, in patients with concomitant somatic diseases, as a result of the use of the improved options of SLOs proposed by us using laparoscopic technologies, the maximum reduction of postoperative complications was achieved.

The use of the improved options of SLOs offered by us, not only compared to traditional operations, but also from other types of SLOs, are technically convenient, precise, thorough execution, the maximum reduction of postoperative complications, patients' mental ease of the operation it is also distinguished by its economic, medical and social advantages.

Thus, patients with concomitant somatic diseases, such as cardiovascular system diseases, anemia, III-IV degrees of obesity, which were previously contraindications for simultaneous surgery, before surgery on abdominal organs performed SLOs in patients with simultaneous surgical pathology found during the intraoperative period, the use of improved original methods laid the groundwork for the successful passage of operations and the expansion of the range of indications for them. It led to the achievement of high economic efficiency due to the reduction of temporary incapacity for work of patients and the reduction of expenses for treatment.

LIST OF REFERENCES

1. Аймагамбетов М. Ж. И Др. Особенности Диагностики И Хирургического Лечения Острого Деструктивного Калькулезного Холецистита У Больных С Избыточной Массой Тела И С Ожирением. Обзор Литературы //Наука И Здравоохранение. – 2019. – №. 3. – С. 54-67.

2. Волков Ю. М. И Др. Сравнительная Характеристика Йединого Лапароскопического (Транспупочного) И Традиционного Лапароскопического Доступа В Лечении Желчно-Каменной Болезни //Актуальные Вопросы Современной Хирургии. – 2018. – С. 30-33.

3. Горбатюк И. Б. Патогенетические Механизмы Взаимно Обремененных Хронического Холецистита, Холестероза Желчного Пузыря С Ожирением И Ишемической Болезнью Сердца //Ветеринарй Ссиенсес. – 2019. – С. 67.

4. Греджев Ф. А. И Др. Острый И Хронический Холециститы. Желчнокаменная Болезнь (Лекция Для Студентов) //Актуальные Вопросы Терапии. – 2016. – С. 7.

5. Замятин В. А., Фаев А. А. Йединый Лапароскопический Доступ В Хирургии Острого Холецистита //Медицина В Кузбассе. – 2014. – №. 1. – С. 12-16.

6. Карабаева В. В., Сидельникова Г. Ф., Колхир В. К. Современная Оценка И Перспективы Применения Сибектана При Лечении Хронического Холецистита В Амбулаторных Условиях //Молодые Ученые И Фармация Xxi Века. – 2015. – С. 449-453.

7. Костырной А. В. И Др. Лапароскопическая Холецистектомия-Отдаленные Результаты //Современные Проблемы Науки И Образования. – 2017. – №. 6. – С. 30-30.

8. Лупсапов А. В. И Др. Лапароскопическая Холецистектомия У Пациентов С Хроническим Калькулезным Холециститом //Аcta Биомедиса Ссиентифиса. – 2005. – №. 3. – С. 310-311.

9. Луцевич О. Е. И Др. Особенности Лапароскопических Операций В Условиях Спаечной Болезни Брюшины И Возможности Йее Лапароскопического Лечения И Профилактики //Тихоокеанский Медицинский Журнал. – 2017. – №. 1. – С. 69-73.

10. Мадьяров В. М., Сахипов М. М., Жапаркулова Г. Р. Диагностика И Хирургическое Лечение Осложненных Форм Холецистолитиаза //Вестник Казахского Национального Медицинского Университета. – 2021. – №. 3. – С. 391-394.

11. Максимов В. А. Хронический Некалькулезный Холецистит И Билиарная Недостаточность //Вопросы Диетологии. – 2015. – Т. 5. – №. 2. – С. 71-78.

12. Маматов Е. А., Закиров Ж. К., Алимбеков Ж. А. Минилапаротомный Доступ В Оперативном Лечении Больных С Острым И Хроническим Холециститом //Наука, Новые Технологии И Инновации Кыргызстана. – 2017. – №. 9. – С. 72-74.

13. Махмадов Ф. И. И Др. Результаты Неотложной Лапароскопической Холецистектомии У Больных С Высоким Операционным Риском //Вестник Авиценны. – 2019. – Т. 21. – №. 1. – С. 121-128.

14. Оревкова О. Д., Галаганова А. А., Стяжкина С. Н. Хронический Холецистит (Клинический Случай) //Вопросы Науки И Образования. – 2017. – №. 11 (12). – С. 209-212.

15. Оревкова О. Д., Галаганова А. А., Стяжкина С. Н. Хронический Холецистит (Клинический Случай) //Вопросы Науки И Образования. – 2017. – №. 11 (12). – С. 209-212.

16. Петрова В. О. Желчнокаменная Болезнь С Развитием Хронического Калькулёзного Холецистита (Клинический Случай) //Форум Молодых Ученых. – 2017. – №. 12. – С. 1453-1457.

17. Полянский И., Андриец В., СХеремет М. Лапароскопическая Холецистектомия У Больной С Полным Обратным Расположением Внутренних Органов //Арта Медиса. – 2015. – №. 1. – С. 50-51.

18. Стяжкина С. Н. И Др. Хронический Калькулезный Холецистит-Актуальное Социально-Економическое Заболевание //Медико-Фармацевтический Журнал «Пулс». – 2016. – Т. 18. – №. 2. – С. 322-326.

19. Кузнецов С.М., Метревели П.Д., Соколова С.В., Толкачев К.С., Салихов Х.Я., Щербатых А.В., Агрызков А.Л., Казанкова О.В., Большешапов А.А. Опыт Применения Ларингеальной Маски При Лапороскопической Холецистектомии // Електронный Научно-Образовательный Вестник "Здоровье И Образование В Ххи Веке". - 2007 Г. -№11. – С. 417.

20. Е.Г. Абдуллаев, М.Ю. Суханов, В.В. Феденко И Др Использование Полипропиленового Сетчатого Ендопротеза При Лечении Больных С Грыжами Передней Брюшной Стенки/.//Ендоскоп. Хир. - 2003. - №5. - С.60-61.

21. Каримов С.И., Назиров Ф.Н., Хаджибаев А.М. К Вопросам Тактики Симултанных Операций При Заболеваниях Органов Брюшной Полости У Лиц Пожилого И Старческого Возраста//Ендоскоп. Хир. - 2003. - №6. - С. 25-26.

22. С.И. Каримов, В.Л. Ким, М.СХ. Хакимов И Др. Малоинвазивные Методы В Лечении Острого Холецистита У Больных С Повышенным Операционным Риском/.//Ендоскоп. Хир. -2003. - №6. - С.35-37.

23. Малоинвазивные Технологии В Диагностике И Лечении Болевой Формы Спаечной Болезни/А.Г. Бебуришвили, И.В. Михин, А.А. Воробьев И Др.//Вестн. Хир. - 2004. - Т.163, №2. - С.38-40.

24. Поиск Альтернативных Путей В Малоинвазивной Оперативной Гинеко- Логии/З.Д. Каримов, К.А. Амиров, Ю.У. Пулатова И Др.//Хирургия Узбекистана. - 2003. - №4. - С.33-37.

25. Пришвин А.П., Майстренко Н.А., Сингаевский С.Б. Оптимизация Методики Лапароскопической Герниопластики//Вестн. Хир. -2003. – Т.162, №6. - С.71-75.

26. Пучков К.В. Использование Полипропиленового Имплантанта В Алло -Пластике Паховых Грыж//Ендоскоп. Хир. - 2003. - №6. - С.15-19.

27. Седов В.М., Стрижелецкий В.В., Гуслев А.Б. Осложнения Ендовидео - Хирургической Герниопластики При Паховых И Бедренных Грыжах//Вестн. Хир . - 2003. - Т.162, №1. - С.80-81.

28. Симултанные Операции В Хирургической Практике/О.С. Олифирова, В.А. Г.В. Омельченко И Др.//Вестн. Хир. - 2002. - Т.161, №5. - С.84-86.

29. Симултанные Операции При Сочетанной Хирургической Патологии/А.Ф. Греджев, В.Ф. СХаталов, Я.Ф. Рогалин И Др.//Клин. Хир. - 2004. - №1. - С. 28-29.

30. Совцов С.А., Пряхин А.Н. Способы Обработки Ложа Желчного Пузыря После Лапароскопической Холецистектомии//Ендоскоп. Хир. - 2003. - №5. - С.48-54.

31. Сочетанные Оперативные Вмешательства В Ендохирургии/А.В. Поташев, В.В. Васильев, Д.Ю. Семенов И Др.//Ендоскоп. Хир. - 2003. - №5. - С.8-12.

32. Сочетанные Лапароскопические Вмешательства При Желчнокаменной Болезни/О.Г. Галимов, М.А. Нуртдинов, Йе.И. Сендерович И Др.//Вестн. Хир. - 2002. - Т.161, №1. - С.82-86.

33. Спаечная Болезнь Брюшной Полости/А.Г. Бебуришвили, А.А. Воробьев, И.В. И Др.//Ендоскоп. Хир. - 2003. - №1. - С.51-63.

34. Сравнительная Оценка Результатов Видео-Лапароскопической, Мини-Лапаротомной И Традиционной Холецистектомии/А.М. Хаджибаев, Ф.Б. Алиджанов, А.Б. Вахидов И Др.//Хирургия Узбекистана. - 2004. - №2. - С.51-53.

35. Хатьков И.Е., Матвеев Н.Л., Гурченкова Й.Ю. Технические Особенности Выполнения Одномоментных Операций При Алиментарно-Конституциональном Ожирении//Ендоскоп. Хир. - 2004. - №3. - С.53-58.

36. Щербеков У.А. Обоснование Малоинвазивных Симултанных Операций В Абдоминальной Хирургии: Дис. ...Канд. Мед. Наук. – Ташкент, 2001. – С. 4-19.

37. Щурыгин С.Н., Дмитриев В.Б. Лечение Спаечной Болезни Брюшной Полости Ендовидеохирургическим Методом//Ендоскоп. Хир. - 2000. - №6. - С.40-41.

38. Економическая Еффективность Внедрения Лапароскопической Холецист- Ектомии У Больных С Желчнокаменной Болезнью/Р.Н. Комаров, Н.В. Комаров, А.С. Маслагин И Др.//Ендоскоп. Хир - 2003. - №4. - С.39-43.Adhesion Formation After Laparoscopic Excision Of Endometriosis And Lysis Of Adhesions/ J.D. Parker, N. Sinaii , J.H. Segars Et Al.//Fertil Steril. – 2005. – Vol.5, №1. – P.61.

39. Introsperative Factors Pedictive Of Failure Of The Ambulatory Regimen After Laparoscopic Cholecysteroctomy//Bueno-Lledo J, Planells-Roig M, Sanahuja-Santafe A. Et Al. Cir Esp. 2005 Sep; 78 (3):168-74.

40. Kulvatunyou N, Schein M.Perforated Subhepatic Appendicitis In The Laparoscopic Era//Surg Endosc. 2001 Jul; 15 (7):769. Epub 2001 May 14.68.

41. Laparoscopic Appendectomy Significantly Reduces Length Of Stay For Perforated Appendicitis//Towfigh S, Chen F, Mason R. Et Al. Surg Endosc. 2006 Jan 25; [Epub Ahead Of Print].

42. Laparoscopic Appendicectomy: Review Of 331 Cases Over 7 Years, In A Saudi Arabian Hospital//Tucker O, Rashid Al-Faqih S, El-Amin O, Zaki A. Endoscopy. 2002 Aug; 34 (8):639-42.

43. Laparoscopic Hernioplasty By Total Extraperitoneal Approach//Alter B, Kuhlmann Hw, Waleczek H, Kozianka J. Zentralbl Chir. 2005 Jun; 130 (3):260-6.

44. Laparoscopic Resection Of A Torsioned Appendix Epiploica In A Previously Appendectomized Patient//Unal E, Yankol Y, Sanal T. Et Al. Surg Laparosc Endosc Percutan Tech. 2005 Dec; 15 (6):371-3.

45. Laparoscopic Versus Standard Appendectomy Outcomes And Cost Comparisons In The Private Sector//Bresciani C, Perez Ro, Habr-Gama A. Et Al. J Gastrointest Surg. 2005 Nov; 9 (8):1174-80.

46. Laparoscopic Surgery For Common Surgical Emergencies: A Population-Based Study//Lam Cm, Yuen Aw, Chik B Et Al.//Surg Endosc. 2005 Jun; 19 (6):774-9. Epub 2005 May 4.

47. Laparoscopy For Abdominal Emergencies: Evidence-Based Guidelines Of The European Association For Endoscopic Surgery//Sauerland S, Agresta F, Bergamaschi R. Et Al. Surg Endosc. 2006 Jan; 20 (1):14-29. Epub 2005 Oct .

48. Laparoscopic Surgical Treatment In Abdominal Emergencies: Personal Experience//Angelini D, Brassetti B, Puce E. Et Al. G Chir. 2002 Apr; 23 (4):151-3.

49. Laparoscopic Versus Conventional Appendectomy: A Prospective Randomized Study//Henle Kp, Beller S, Rechner J. Et Al. Chirurg. 1996 May; 67 (5):526-30.

50. Laparoscopic Cholecystectomy In Non-Lithiasis Cholecystopathies//Bradea C, Niculescu D, Plesa C. Et Al. Rev Med Chir Soc Med Nat Iasi. 2000 Oct-Dec; 104 (4):91-3.

51. 197. Laparoscopy In Abdominal Emergencies. Indications And Limitations/S.G. Perri, F. Altilia, F. Pietrangeli Et Al.//Chir Ital. 2002 Mar-Apr;54(2):165-78.

52. 198. Laparoscopic Cholecystectomy In Patients With Previous Upper Or Lower Abdominal Surgery/A.J. Karayiannakis, A. Polychronidis, S. Perente Et Al.//Surg Endosc. 2004 Jan; 18 (1):97-101. Epub 2003 Oct 23.

53.

54. Popovic J, Sulovic V, Vucetic D.Laparoscopy Treatment Of Adnexal Sterility//Clin Exp Obstet Gynecol. 2005; 32 (1):31-4.Clinic Of Gynecology And Obstetrics.

55. Randomized Clinical Trial Of The Effect Of Preoperative Dexamethasone On Nausea And Vomiting After Laparoscopic Cholecystectomy/C.V. Feo, D. Sortini, R. Ragazzi Et Al.//Br J Surg. 2006. –Vol. 9, №2. – R.123-124.

56. 223. Shayani V.Laparoscopic Adhesiolysis In Patients With Chronic Abdominal Pain//Lancet. - 2003. – Vol.28, №6. – R.243.

57. Tanovic H, Mesihovic R, Muhovic S. Randomized Trial Of Tep Laparoscopic Hernioplasty Versus Bassni Inguinal Hernia Repair//Med Arh. – 2005. – Vol.59, №4. – R.214-216.

58. The Development Of Laparoscopic Surgery In Spain/X. Feliu, E.M. Targarona, A. Garcia-Agusti Et Al.//Dig Surg. – 2004. – Vol.21, №5. – R. 421-425. 102.

59. The Therapeutic Value Of Elective Laparoscopic Appendectomy In The Management Of Chronic Abdominal Pain/S.V. Hosseini, M. Haghbeen, H. Yarmohammadi Et Al.//Saudi Med J. – 2005. – Vol.26, №9. – R.82-83. 103.

60. Tittel A, Schumpelick V. Laparoscopic Surgery: Expectations And Reality//Chirurg. – 2001. Vol.72, №3. – 35-37.

61. <u>Tiwari A</u>, <u>Peters J.L</u>. Laparoscopic Adhesiolysis In Patients With Chronic Abdominal Pain//<u>Lancet.</u> 2003. - Vol.28, №3. – P.43-44.

62. Transvaginal Three-Dimensional Ultrasonography Combined With Serum Ca 125 Level For The Diagnosis Of Pelvic Adhesions Before Laparoscopic Surgery/K.M. <u>Seow</u>, Y.H. <u>Lin</u>, B.C. <u>Hsieh</u> Et Al.//<u>J Am Assoc Gynecol Laparosc.</u> – 2003. – Vol.10, №3. P.320-326.

63. <u>Utpal D</u>. Laparoscopic Versus Open Appendectomy In West Bengal, India//<u>Chin J Dig Dis.</u> – 2005. – Vol. 6, №4. - P. 165-169.

64. Ćwik G. Et Al. The Value Of Percutaneous Ultrasound In Predicting Conversion From Laparoscopic To Open Cholecystectomy Due To Acute Cholecystitis //Surgical Endoscopy. – 2013. – Vol. 27. – Pp. 2561-2568.

65. Ding L. Et Al. Oral Administration Of Nanoiron Sulfide Supernatant For The Treatment Of Gallbladder Stones With Chronic Cholecystitis //Acs Applied Bio Materials. – 2020. – Vol. 4. – №. 5. – Pp. 3773-3785.

66. Inoue T. Et Al. Long-Term Outcomes Of Endoscopic Gallbladder Stenting In High-Risk Surgical Patients With Calculous Cholecystitis (With Videos) //Gastrointestinal Endoscopy. – 2016. – Vol. 83. – №. 5. – Pp. 905-913.

67. Koti R. S., Davidson C. J., Davidson B. R. Surgical Management Of Acute Cholecystitis //Langenbeck's Archives Of Surgery. – 2015. – Vol. 400. – Pp. 403-419.

68. Kwaan M. R. Et Al. Abdominoperineal Resection, Pelvic Exenteration, And Additional Organ Resection Increase The Risk Of Surgical Site Infection After Elective Colorectal Surgery: An American College Of Surgeons National Surgical Quality Improvement Program Analysis //Surgical Infections. – 2015. – Vol. 16. – №. 6. – Pp. 675-683.

69. Mahoney R. C. Et Al. Enormous Gallstone Discovered In The Setting Of Acute-On-Chronic Cholecystitis //Hawai'i Journal Of Health & Social Welfare. – 2021. – Vol. 80. – №. 11 Suppl 3. – Pp. 38.

70. Matsumura T. Et Al. Closure Of The Cystic Duct Orifice In Laparoscopic Subtotal Cholecystectomy For Severe Cholecystitis //Asian Journal Of Endoscopic Surgery. – 2018. – Vol. 11. – №. 3. – Pp. 206-211.

71. Orr N. T., Davenport D. L., Roth J. S. Outcomes Of Simultaneous Laparoscopic Cholecystectomy And Ventral Hernia Repair Compared To That Of Laparoscopic Cholecystectomy Alone //Surgical Endoscopy. – 2013. – Vol. 27. – Pp. 67-73.

72. SIMULTANEOUS LAPAROSCOPIC OPERATIONS IN HIGH RISK PATIENTS - Ismailov U.S., Batirov D.Y., Rakhimov A.P., Allanazarov A.K., Umarov Z.Z., Sheniyazov S.S., Rojobov R.R. 58-70

73. The factor analysis of the results of modern treatment of patients with liver cirrhosis with portal hypertension. Astana Medical Journal, 116, 2023, 30-34. MS Khakimov, UI Matkuliev, DY Batirov, ZZ Umarov, AX Allanazarov, AP Rakhimov.

74. Simultan Laparoskopik Operatsiyalarni Surunkali Kamqonlik Kuzatilgan Bemorlarda O'Tkazilish Natijalarini Yaxshilash // Batirov D.Y., Allanazarov A.X., Raximov A.P., Sheniyazov SH., Rojobov, Qo'ziyeva Sh.Sh // International Journal of Economy and Innovation |Volume 32| Gospodarka i Innowacje 90

75. Minimally Invasive Interventions in Portal Hypertension Complication with Esophageal and Gastric Varicose Veins. Maktkuliev O'tkirbek Ismailovich, Batirov Davronbek Yusupovich, Umarov Zafarbek Zaripbaevich, Allanazarov Allanazar Khudashkurovich, Rakhimov Anvarbek Pulatovich, Nurmatov Sirojbek Tajibaevich - Scholastic: Journal of Natural and Medical Education, 2023.

76. Improving the results of simultaneous laparoscopic surgery in patients with chronic deficiency. DY Batirov, Allanazarov A Kh, AP Rakhimov, RR Rojobov - European journal of modern medicine and practice, 2023

www.ingramcontent.com/pod-product-compliance
Lightning Source LLC
Chambersburg PA
CBHW060750260726
48660CB00002B/557